En

The Sports Lover's Guide to Recovery

Although his profession is elsewhere, in this book Andrew Dieden is also a teacher. Andy teaches (or, if you prefer, coaches) with authority. He knows both worlds of which he speaks and the connection between the two. Just read the preface. He doesn't have to say much more about where he has been. Like a good coach's locker room talk when losing the game at halftime, he spends most of his time talking about what the team can do and where the team is going, not where the team has been. The rest of the book is about what his intended audience can do and achieve, if they train hard and pay attention. It's about a better game of life.

When Andy coaches, he trains people in body and spirit to leave behind a negative and reach a positive way of life. His message, while cast in a huge sports metaphor, is a message of living for anyone struggling with life's difficulties, and it is a message cast in plain language. It is the message of one who "has walked in your shoes."

The sports metaphor is more than a clever trick to get the reader's attention. Andy Dieden truly finds life lessons in every sport and presents them to the sports-loving recovering alcoholic as life principles. Read closely the introductions to each chapter. All are life lessons as seen through the eyes and thoughts of athletes and their coaches.

A worthy book to write and very much worth the read.

—John E. Ingersoll
Director, Bureau of Narcotics
and Dangerous Drugs (today's DEA),
1968–1973

As a golf pro, I often hear people comparing playing golf to living life. I believe the comparison is valid. As is true of many sports, golf tests our virtues, such as integrity, cooperation, honesty, humility, and dedication. The game also exposes weaknesses that we can work on to build confidence and self-esteem. I believe that's why golf's lessons are so popular.

This book takes the lessons one learns in sports and applies them to addiction, a disease that affects everyone in one way or another. In this book, the problem and the solution are clearly presented in an inviting, motivational way. The insightful quotes from sports legends, along with the historical sports stories, provide concrete examples that Andrew Dieden uses as a basis for explaining how the principles of recovery work. He has found an entertaining way to present a very serious topic. Regardless of whether you struggle with addiction or not, *The Sports Lover's Guide to Recovery* will help you better understand recovery and improve your level of play. The book scores a birdie!

> —Mark Cato
> Former PGA tour player, PGA professional

The Sports Lover's Guide to Recovery is remarkable, managing to treat its compelling subject with all the seriousness it deserves while providing optimism, inspiration, and humor throughout. Starting with a revelation that demonstrates that the author knows of what he writes, Mr. Dieden supplies the building blocks for recovery through motivating sports metaphors, incorporating tales of victory over the odds into realistic steps for triumphing over a powerful addiction. Whether one is a sports neophyte such as myself or a seasoned aficionado, this book is a must-read for anyone trying to preserve his or her relationship, job, or life from the devastation of addiction.

> —Hon. Virginia A. Mellema, Ph.D.
> U.S. Federal Administrative Judge, EEOC

THE SPORTS LOVER'S
GUIDE TO RECOVERY

THE SPORTS LOVER'S GUIDE TO RECOVERY

*Strategies and
Rules of the Game*

■ ■ ■

Andrew L. Dieden

*"If you live long enough,
lots of nice things happen."*

➤ George Halas, Pro Football
Hall of Fame coach and owner

HAZELDEN

Hazelden
Center City, Minnesota 55012-0176
1-800-328-0094
1-651-213-4590 (Fax)
hazelden.org

Library of Congress Cataloging-in-Publication Data
Dieden, Andrew L.
    The sports lover's guide to recovery : strategies and rules of
the game / by Andrew L. Dieden.
        p. cm.
    Includes bibliographical references.
    ISBN 978-1-59285-485-1 (softcover)
    1. Substance abuse—Treatment. 2. Addicts—Rehabilitation.
3. Athletes—Rehabilitation. 4. Sports—Miscellanea. I. Title.
    HV4998.D54 2008
    616.86'03—dc22

                                            2007039738

11 10 09 08   1 2 3 4 5 6

Cover design by David Spohn
Interior design and typesetting by
    BookMobile Design & Publishing Services

For Mom and Dad

*The two greatest coaches and fans
I can imagine.*

Contents

■ ■ ■

*"Courage is not the absence of fear,
but simply moving on with dignity
despite that fear."*

➤ Pat Riley,
champion NBA player and coach

Foreword

■ ■ ■

*"If you don't like the way
things are going, change the way
you're doing things."*

➤ Jim Sweeney,
college football head coach

Addiction affects people in different ways. It can
manifest itself through an excess of drugs and alcohol, work, food, gambling, or sex. Whatever form it
takes, addiction is the compulsive attempt to gen-
erate or abolish a feeling. Often this feeling stems
from the core belief that one is not good enough.
Addicts consistently try to find ways to prove that
they are good enough and with equal consistency
try to avoid feeling that they are not. Despite the
negative consequences associated with addiction,
addicts will continue to engage in destructive behaviors in a desperate attempt to find temporary
solutions to chronic problems. Unfortunately, the
solution of addiction soon becomes the problem
and masks the core problems that really need to be
looked at.

To identify these problems, addicts must find ways to recovery from addiction. The concept of recovery can seem overwhelming due to the multitude of opinions of how it should be done and each addict's beliefs about what it means to be in recovery. It is only when addicts feel that recovery is relevant to their lives that real change is possible. Recovery becomes a reality when addicts believe that what they want is something that they can have.

First, addicts must learn to identify what is not working for them. Part of what is so difficult for addicts is verbalizing what it is they want or need. They have learned to communicate how they feel through their behaviors. The first goal is to identify how the addict feels and then to help him to find the words to communicate the feelings.

Once the addict is able to identify what he is feeling, then he can choose an alternative to the temporary solution of drinking, using, or acting out, something that might actually serve as a permanent solution to a chronic problem. The frustration for most addicts is that the alternative solution generally takes longer than the instant gratification a drug or impulsive behavior has to offer. For the new behavior to have a chance of working, addicts need to feel a certain sense of movement and reward, along with a sense of hope.

What Andrew Dieden has written on the following pages gives me a sense of hope that learning about recovery will be less intimidating and more relatable. Almost everyone will relate to the stories in this book. The emotions associated with winning, losing, discipline, and surrender are universal, even if you're not a sports fan.

There is nothing more intimidating, exhilarating, disappointing, and rewarding than the game of life. The same can be said of sports and the process of recovery. Both sports and recovery require a person to exercise discipline, courage, and some form of surrender. The stories in this book illustrate how athletes and addicts must acknowledge their weaknesses in order to achieve their greatest successes. Andrew Dieden has found a way to make the idea of recovery less intimidating, even to those who might not be ready to stop drinking or using. He has written a book that has found a fun and manageable way to address a serious topic. Due to the captivating sports stories, you may actually forget that you are reading a book about recovery, a book that can help you save your life.

—Dr. Joanna M. Ceppi, Psychologist,
Promises Treatment Center,
Malibu, California

Preface

■ ■ ■

*"Coaching that team is like having a
window seat on the Hindenburg."*

➤ Bob Plager,
NHL hockey player

If you or someone you know is anything like I was
during the last years of my drinking, you're hitting
the booze or drugs hard. You and your life are a
mess. You fear your future if you continue to drink
but can't imagine life without drinking. You've run
up against a tough opponent and may be thinking
to yourself, "If I can just tackle this problem, I can
get back on top of things." This guide's purpose is to
assure you that you *can* get back on top of things. In
the tennis match of life, however, your drinking or
using has probably caused you to drop a few games
or maybe even a set. This does not mean that you
have lost the match. You can still win if you adjust
the way you're playing.

■ ■ ■

"Don't ever wrestle with a pig.
You'll both get dirty, but only the
pig will enjoy it."

━ Cale Yarborough,
champion NASCAR driver

Before I took my last drink, I was like an older ballplayer who had never taken care of himself at the end of a long season. I felt physically run down, and I was mentally troubled by shame and remorse, a lost soul. Being the man that I was, I had ended my umpteenth relationship by not answering her phone calls. I was drinking booze and chewing tobacco like a madman. I *was* a madman. Very near the end, after a New Year's binge in Chicago, I was denied admission onto my connecting flight out of Arizona that was to take me home to California. I was too drunk.

I decided to make the most of being too drunk to fly by going out on the town. I ended up smoking weed on a fire escape in a ghetto with a couple of strippers. The strippers stole my wallet and luggage, including my return ticket. When I reported the mugging to the police, they wanted to hook me up to some machines in order to monitor my sleep. You see, the police were doing research on alcoholic sleeping patterns. When I refused, they turned me out. In turn, I threw up in front of the officers.

I walked through the desert all night to the airport. The clock was running down, and I was out of time-outs. I knew that the game was lost the way I was playing it. I desperately needed a new game. I had to stop drinking and get in shape for life.

■ ■ ■

"We all get 24 hours each day.
That's the only fair thing; it's the only
thing that's equal. What we do with
those 24 hours is up to us."

➤ Sam Huff,
Pro Football Hall of Fame linebacker

In order to acquire the strength, flexibility, endurance, and balance necessary to beat alcohol, I faithfully adopted a multiple-exercise program that millions of alcoholics and addicts have proven successful. I have stuck with the program and work it every day as well as I can. My fight against booze is too important for me to skip any exercises. My life is at stake.

If you love sports, you will understand more quickly and easily the apparent nonsense everyone in recovery seems to be preaching by associating recovery with ideas that you already know. In this guide, I use sports terms, concepts, quotes, and stories to show how I approach the basics of my recovery program. Using these analogies can help you learn and execute a winning strategy in an easier, more meaningful way.

The game here is addiction, and we win by living our lives happily and comfortably with the affliction. It may sound obvious, but living your life happily and comfortably without alcohol and drugs means that you will be happy and comfortable. You *can* be happy.

For me, happiness was why I got drunk. Getting drunk initially made me happier, so I kept doing it. Eventually, alcohol didn't work anymore. In fact, it actually prevented me from being happy. I made this significant discovery only after I had stopped drinking for a while.

At the end of my drinking, there were two teams remaining that were willing to offer me a contract: Uncontrollable Drinking and Recovery. As a free agent, I could make the choice. Uncontrollable Drinking promised suffering, followed by death. Recovery offered a chance to live happily. Although less appealing, Uncontrollable Drinking was more familiar to me. I knew the players and the rules. But reluctantly I decided to sign on with Recovery.

My Recovery contract contained several terms and conditions that initially made me think twice.

Still, I didn't have much of a choice. Thanks in part to those terms and conditions, I am now, after only a short time, living happily and comfortably without booze. I believe any alcoholic or addict can do the same. It may help to think of sobriety as the ball; we need to gain possession and, once we do, we must protect it.

In this book, I use the terms "alcohol" and "drugs" interchangeably because alcohol is a drug. Alcoholics are drug addicts. Alcoholics and other drug addicts have the same disease—addiction.

Also, I use primarily the male pronoun "him," for simplicity. I do not intend any discrimination. Neither the sports-lover class nor the addict class is exclusive of either gender. Women and men, on an equal basis, are members of both classes.

Acknowledgments

■ ■ ■

"You gotta be a grinder."

— Chris Spielman, NFL linebacker

One of the great things sobriety offers is the chance to pass it on, which is the reason I wrote this book. My sobriety couldn't have happened in the first place without a program and a support system. So, in a very real sense, this book has been possible because of the team on which I am grateful to play.

My team includes my family, friends, fellows, colleagues, people who have helped me with this project, and a handful of individuals who planted seeds that grew into recovery. You have all been more than I deserve. I am indebted to every one of you for helping me regain and develop my soul. Passing on what you've given me is part of my effort to repay you.

To my family, especially my parents, Walt and Sue (and stepfather, Howard); siblings Jeff (and Melinda), Shelley, and Matt; nieces Elise, Laura, and Marie; Aunt Sally (and Uncle Richard); cousins Michael, Terri, Kate, Bill, Libby, Ed (and Kathy), Jonathan, Dick, and Beverly (and Bob); the Ichinagas; and those unnamed:

You have never let me doubt that I would be loved without reservation. I have caused you all anxiety about my well-being and a lot of embarrassment, which I sincerely regret. I love you all. Thank you.

To my friends, especially Bill (The Bird) Fairey and Alex (and my second parents, Bill Sr. and Sue), Jamal and Cece, Rocky and Chris, Gal and Janelle, Bruce and Kelly, Shark and K.Z., Grube and Tracy, Andrew and Angie, Lar, Kev and Tricia, Antonio, Ricardo and Kelli, Chip and Cindy, Johnny and Janice, Pick and Barbara, Todd and Pam, Proc and Erin, Hugh and Connie, Bob K., Bob S., Bob L., Brenda, and those unnamed: You made it abundantly clear that it was okay, indeed preferable, if I didn't party anymore. I love you all. Thank you.

To my fellows, especially my patient and wise sponsor, Leon; the Friday Night Larkspur group; and the Marin and San Francisco fellowships: You continually show and teach me that happiness comes when we do a few simple, sometimes challenging things. Thank you all. I am sincerely grateful.

To the people who let me know the truth before I was willing to make a change, particularly Bob Montgomery who told me that all I cared about was in the beer can I was holding; the boy on the football field who asked if I was a good person; the stranger I fought at a party who exclaimed in disgust, "Look at you!"; and Julie, who told me in a matter-of-fact way that I was an alcoholic twelve years before I stopped drinking: Your comments were honest, insightful, and correct. I hope I never forget them. Thank you.

To those who encouraged and helped me write this book, especially my informal editors (Jack Ingersoll, Jeff Dieden, Michael Dieden, Michael Kaye, Kristine Van Dorsten, Matt Dieden, Leon Abrams, Lee Rosenthal, Matt Sullivan, Dr. Brigitte Lank, Dr. Joanna M. Ceppi, Jeannette Boudreau, Clayton Parker, Troy Vukovich, Mark Cato, Steve McAllister, and the Hon. Virginia Mellema), and to the many others who have provided valuable lessons and feedback, including Franco Erspamer: Good ideas often don't count for much without being developed and refined. Thanks for your help.

I'd like to thank especially the accomplished and talented Dr. Joanna M. Ceppi, who took time away from her busy life to write the foreword, a major contribution to this book. Also, thanks to my fellow members on the National Council on Alcoholism and other Drug Addictions–Bay Area (NCADA-BA) board, and the other individuals who have endorsed this book: Your willingness to come forward and address a largely unspoken epidemic is admirable, and I sincerely appreciate it.

Thank you to Jeff Tedford, University of California football head coach, for giving his time and thoughts on the book, coaching, and life in general. Thanks also to his staff, Coach Michalczik, Coach McHugh, and Athletic Director Sandy Barbour and her staff. The book is much better because of each of you. Thanks also to the athletes and coaches whom I've been privileged to watch, hear, and read about throughout my life, especially those quoted and referenced in this book. Chris Spielman's quote that heads this acknowledgment hit home with me in early sobriety and still keeps me going during tough times. Thanks also to the members of the Team Hamana mountain bike team.

A loving thanks to Kristine (and Zoe) who motivated me to work through adversity and find the right publisher. You were right. It worked out very well. Working with Hazelden Publishing—Don Freeman, Becky Post, Karen Chernyaev, April Dahl, David Spohn, and all the other talented, committed people there—has been an incredible creative experience.

For those I've failed to mention, please chalk it up to years of excessive drinking, not any intention to snub you. I apologize.

PLAY BALL

*"Do you know what my favorite
part of the game is? The opportunity
to play. It is as simple as that. God,
I love that opportunity."*

➤ Mike Singletary,
Pro Football Hall of Fame linebacker

No one has ever run like the "Kansas Comet," Chicago Bears running back Gale Sayers. Sayers eluded tacklers with breathtaking speed, cutting ability, and gracefulness. In 1965, he scored six touchdowns in a single game on his way to Rookie of the Year honors. He is the all-time kickoff return leader and the youngest player ever inducted into the Pro Football Hall of Fame. Sayers's path to football immortality, however, was not easy.

In 1968, Sayers ripped his knee apart. In a game against the 49ers, he took the ball and ran around the end, following his blockers toward the sideline. Kermit Alexander, 49ers' cornerback, approached to make the tackle. As Sayers planted his outside foot to cut back toward the center of the field, Alexander dove at Sayers's leg with his shoulder, hitting Sayers's knee hard.

With his foot stuck in the turf and his momentum moving forward, there was nowhere for Sayers's knee to go except sideways, bending ninety degrees in a direction it was never intended to bend. Sayers momentarily passed out. His medial collateral ligament, medial meniscus, and anterior cruciate ligament were all torn. Some thought that the Kansas Comet had played his last down as a running back.

Dr. Theodore Fox, the Bears' bone specialist, told Sayers that his knee was gone. Understandably, Sayers's first reaction was fear and self-pity. "Why me, why did it have to be me?" he thought to himself. "And then I put my head in my hands and started to cry." This attitude didn't last long, though. "As soon as I got out of the hospital I more or less accepted my injury and determined to get my knee back in shape so that I could play the next year. . . ." Sayers recalled, ". . . and not because I was out to prove anything to anybody else . . . everything I try to prove is to myself."

With the help of many people, including his wife, Linda, and his great friend and roommate, Brian Piccolo, Sayers worked tirelessly and accomplished the improbable. In the first game of 1969, the man wearing number forty, the Kansas Comet, returned the opening kickoff sixty-nine yards. He went on to lead the league in rushing that year. Commenting on the 1969 season, Sayers said, ". . . if you work hard enough, if you're willing to endure the pain, if you're willing to sacrifice yourself, you can make it back right away." Sayers was voted the NFL's Most Courageous Player in 1970. He humbly dedicated the award to Piccolo.

Sayers did not let the fear of what might happen deter him from moving forward with his life. Although he had no idea whether he'd be able to play again, Sayers completely committed himself to his recovery. Fueled by others' encouragement and enthusiasm, and his own complete desire, Sayers put in all the hard work required to make progress. His progress told him that returning to the game was possible, which fueled an even greater daily effort. In the end, he experienced success with benefits far beyond his personal return to the gridiron.

Sayers's recovery enriched not only his life but many others' lives as well. It allowed him to help his team win. It also brought joy to his fans and validation to legendary Bears owner George Halas, who believed in Sayers when many did not.

The amazing thing is that, while Sayers's story is genuinely remarkable in football, it is not by any means without parallel or unusual in the world of addiction. Similar stories occur all the time in recovery. Millions of us in recovery have shown great courage and resolve by accepting our situation, putting our fears aside, making a complete commitment, and working hard to overcome what initially seemed like impossible odds.

Accepting our situation means acknowledging that something is wrong with us that requires us to take action. Contrary to a once-popular misconception, being an addict doesn't mean that something is "wrong" with us in a moral sense. What *is* wrong is that our reaction to alcohol and drugs is simply different from most people's reaction.

Unlike most people, when addicts experience repeated alcohol- or drug-related negative consequences, we continue to see drinking or using drugs as an option. This allows our minds to return to alcohol and drugs, and at some point, we start up again, taking that first drink or drug. Then, after taking the first, our craving for more overpowers our willpower to stop. Thus, we cannot choose to stop once we have started, and we suffer even more negative consequences.

Gaining the ability to not take the first drink or drug is the key. In order to do so, we need to commit ourselves to learning and playing a new game, a game with different rules, different thinking, and different behaviors than the addiction game to which we have grown accustomed.

In this guide, we'll cover the rules of the sobriety game and the strategies for winning our recovery. We'll start by covering our commitment to a positive, productive lifestyle. Next, we'll discuss the training program that makes us fit enough to execute that lifestyle. Finally, we'll see how to maintain our fitness in order to continue living our useful, happy, and contented lives.

Of course, any genuine commitment requires that we address the fear that can hold us back. It requires dispensing our trepidation about the future, such as worries about what we will become and what our lives in recovery will be like. Few of us starting out in recovery want to be the stereotypical sober addict, the beat-up guy in a trench coat with a cup of coffee and a burning smoke. Don't worry, if that's not who you want to be, that's not who you'll become. Tragically, many addicts continue drinking and using because we fear that a recovery program will brainwash us into becoming nothing more than drones.

The fear of being brainwashed should not concern anyone who is considering recovery. Our different backgrounds, skills, abilities, problems, and needs make each of our paths to recovery unique. Recovery is simply a way of improving ourselves by adopting, deleting, maximizing, and minimizing elements of life that, in the right combinations, allow happiness. Making the improvements happen requires a lot of effort, but we don't have to do it by ourselves. We should take heart in the fact that we will receive plenty of help along the way.

■ ■ ■

"Don't be afraid if things seem difficult in the beginning. That's only the initial impression. The important thing is not to retreat; you have to master yourself."

➤ Olga Korbut,
four-time Olympic gold medal gymnast

The strength we receive from others' encouragement and enthusiasm, as well as our own complete desire to live healthfully again, will allow us to make progress. Our progress will then show us that our recovery is possible, which will empower us to make an even greater daily effort. Playing our new game will soon seem natural to us, and we'll wonder why we ever lived any other way. We'll experience enlightenment while avoiding disaster.

A countless number of us in recovery, upon seeing clearly how we had been living our lives, say to ourselves, "If I had continued drinking and using, I would have lost it all." "Losing it all" means losing not just what we have accomplished and accumulated; it means losing the opportunity our future holds. This is why the saying Vince Lombardi made famous is directly applicable to addicts: "Winning isn't everything; it's the only thing."

Winning our recovery isn't easy, but the benefits are well worth the effort. Like Gale Sayers's recovery from knee surgery, when we help ourselves recover from addiction, we help not only ourselves; we help others—the people we love, the people who have stuck with us, and the world. Yes, even people we don't know benefit from our recovery. And, if we don't work toward recovery, we will continue devastating and perhaps killing ourselves, the people we love, and the people around us.

Let's face it, the last thing our world needs is another cancer in the clubhouse. Let's follow the Kansas Comet's example by setting our fear aside, completely committing ourselves to recovery, training consistently, and maintaining our fitness. Let's prove to ourselves that we can do it. If we do, we will have happy, purposeful lives that we'll want to share. We'll know contentment we never even imagined.

If that's what *you* want, you're ready to seize the opportunity to play ball again. You're ready to start winning again. Like many things in life, thinking about recovery is harder than actually doing it. Rather than engaging in the torturous game of fear-inducing mental gymnastics, it's easier to simply start the process by accepting our situation and completely committing ourselves to recovery.

■ ■ ■

"I am a survivor, not a victim."

➤ Lance Armstrong, cancer survivor,
seven-time Tour de France champion

COMMITMENT:
THE RECOVERY CONTRACT

*"Never let your head hang down.
Never give up and sit down and
grieve. Find another way."*

— Satchel Paige,
National Baseball Hall of Fame pitcher

In 2005, race car rookie Danica Patrick drove her car 230 miles per hour, the fastest practice speed of the month for Indianapolis 500 (Indy) qualifying. She went on to post the fourth-fastest qualifying time and finished fourth overall in the most famous car race in the world. Along the way, Patrick made history.

Car racing is a sport dominated by men. With few exceptions, female participation has been limited to ownership, being a fan, or modeling next to the cars. When she was young, none of these options interested Patrick. "Racing was my focus and my sole desire." She refused to be limited by past practice. Although she was not the first woman to race at Indy (three women had done it before), she was the first woman ever to lead the race, which she did for nineteen laps. She had a good chance to win, but with eleven laps to go, low fuel made her slow down in order to finish the race. Today she's hungrier than ever to realize her dream—winning the Indy checkered flag.

People around the globe have fallen in love with Patrick for her driving ability, her heart, and her intelligence. When she first raced at Indy, the TV coverage received a 40 percent spike in ratings. Still, novelty wears off quickly if it isn't followed by substance. Fans, team owners, and sponsors don't stick around without race results.

Patrick hasn't taken solace in the fact that she almost won Indy or that she was named 2005 Rookie of the Year. She races to win. "You don't ever want to have excuses, because that means there's a reason you didn't win." In other words, she doesn't look for reasons to lose. After a successful 2006, in which she finished as the twelfth-fastest driver overall, Patrick was named the March of Dimes New York Chapter Sportswoman of the Year. Her popularity has steadily increased since her 2005 Indy appearance.

Her popularity with race fans also makes her

popular with sponsors. In addition to her race team and its sponsors, a short list of her endorsements includes Bell Helmets, XM Radio, Hostess Cakes, and Motorola. Obviously, all of these deals involve contracts, and every contract she signs requires her commitment.

Contracts are a part of life. So is commitment. Contracts and commitments are a privilege. They offer the opportunity for devotion and reward. This is true for athletes, and it's also true for recovering addicts.

■ ■ ■

"The more difficult the victory,
the greater the happiness in winning."

➥ Pelé
(Edson Arantes do Nascimento),
World Cup soccer champion

Professional athletes and recovering addicts each have contracts that contain unique terms and conditions. Athletes enter into team and sponsorship contracts, while recovering addicts enter into contracts with themselves, their own spiritual foundation, and others in recovery. In each case, the contract identifies what is being exchanged in the deal.

The typical professional sports contract provides

what the player will be paid. In exchange, the player commits to clauses related to participation in sports, collective bargaining, merchandising rights, and ethics. These terms and conditions are prerequisites to compensation. If the player fails to meet them, he forfeits his pay.

Recovering addicts' contracts provide the opportunity to live happily without booze and other drugs. Of course, there are prerequisites in those contracts as well. The first prerequisite is our acknowledgment that rules, in fact, exist and that the rules apply directly to us.

Recovery's most fundamental rule is to live by the truth at all times. Our commitment does not stop there. Our contracts also require that we

- accept guidance from a coach;
- admit that alcohol and/or drugs have made a mess out of our lives;
- have faith that a force with power beyond ours will help us live happily without alcohol and drugs;
- put others' (our teams') interests before our own.

If we fail to play by these simple rules, we forfeit our opportunity to live happily. And our contracts don't change as our lives improve. We must continually remind ourselves that without our commitment to these rules, any progress we've made will be lost. Fortunately, in case we forget, we have a coach to remind us.

THE COACH

*"It is what you learn after
you know it all that counts."*

➤ John Wooden,
Basketball Hall of Fame college coach

During the Cold War era, communist Europe was home to many of the world's greatest athletes. Although they were celebrities in the communist world, few of us would recognize them by name because their governments didn't permit them to compete in capitalist events, other than at the Olympics. Some of the truly exceptional athletes from behind the Iron Curtain were well-known in the free world, however. One of these truly exceptional athletes was Polish mountain climber, Wanda Rutkiewicz.

Mountains were her great escape. Rutkiewicz grew up in war-torn Poland just after World War II, and her childhood was tough. First, her little brother was blown up by a land mine while playing in the rubble of a bombed house. Later, her father was axed to

death, then buried in the family garden. These trag-
edies left Wanda afraid of people.

While she may have feared people, Rutkiewicz was
certainly not afraid of heights or physical exertion.
She is widely considered the greatest female mountain climber ever to live. A climber's success is often
measured by reaching the summit of the world's tall-
est mountains, known as the "Eight-Ks"—those that
stand at least eight thousand meters above sea level
(that's more than five miles, straight up). In her lifetime, Wanda climbed eight of the world's fourteen
Eight-Ks.

In 1978, Rutkiewicz became the first European
woman to reach the summit of Mount Everest. In
1986, without using bottled oxygen, she became the
first woman to climb K2, the world's second-tallest
mountain but a much more difficult climb than
Everest. That year, thirteen people died trying to
reach K2's summit. Some were blown off by wind,
some fell, and a 125-miles-per-hour avalanche killed
others. But Rutkiewicz made it.

She was simply an incredible climber. Although
she was only 5'5" tall, she was remarkably strong. She
was known to win arm-wrestling matches, one after
another, against supposedly stronger male climbers.
She also trained hard, developing great technique
and balance. More than anything, Rutkiewicz was
determined.

The feeling of reaching a difficult summit has been compared to alcohol and drug addiction, triggering a dopamine release that some climbers crave again and again. This may explain Rutkiewicz's determination to overcome any obstacle in order to reach the world's toughest summits. Unfortunately, it was her insatiable drive that eventually caused her death.

Although the Polish climbers are renowned as great "team" climbers, this wasn't always true of Rutkiewicz. By 1992, her independence had alienated many of her fellow climbers. To make matters worse, many of her friends had already retired from climbing or were dead. Rutkiewicz was a lonely woman when she set off to climb Kangchenjunga, the world's third-tallest mountain and the only Eight-K never climbed by a woman.

The climb started well, but soon four of the six climbers had to turn back. Only Rutkiewicz and young Carlos Carsolio were able to make a final summit attempt. When her climbing slowed, Rutkiewicz ordered Carsolio to go ahead, leaving both to climb solo. Eventually, Carsolio lost sight of Rutkiewicz and reached the summit. On his way down, it was getting dark, and he was almost out of water and food. He had to hurry. When Carsolio came across Rutkiewicz, she was huddled in a small ice hole, trying to escape the harsh weather. She, too, was low on food and water. Carsolio suggested she climb down with him.

"No, no, I will be okay," she said. "I'm just cold. Once the sun comes up, I will be warm and go for the summit."

This was insanity. He asked Rutkiewicz to reconsider. She would not. Carsolio was the last person to see or hear from Rutkiewicz. She died alone, cold, five miles high, insisting that she knew what she was doing. She died the death of an addict, determined to feel that elusive high one more time.

With drug and alcohol addiction, a recovery rookie is like a mountain climber who wants to conquer a new peak. Mountain climbers are taught not to climb alone because it isn't safe. Similarly, recovery rookies shouldn't assault addiction by themselves.

If we attempt to get sober solo, we may learn for ourselves the hard, potentially deadly lessons that a sponsor could have taught us without the risk of injury. A sponsor will guide us past the difficult sections that have endangered and killed many addicts in the past. Addiction is every bit as dangerous as mountain climbing. In fact, historically, far more people have died from addiction than from mountain climbing. While a mountain climber may die a relatively quick, pain-free death, a practicing addict typically suffers long and hard before the blessing of death arrives. If we value our lives and those we love, we'll get ourselves a good guide.

■ ■ ■

*"The best and fastest way
to learn a sport is to watch
and imitate a champion."*

— Jean-Claude Killy,
three-time Olympic gold medal skier

A sponsor is like a climbing guide or a coach. He is our main sobriety mentor, an addict who has done what is necessary to live happily without booze and dope. He continues doing these things because if he doesn't, he will drink or use again. We can trust our sponsor because he has been in our shoes and because guiding rookies helps him continue his own winning lifestyle.

Upon entering recovery, we choose a sponsor we want to emulate. In choosing a sponsor, some people look for common life experiences. Others look for someone who has an attitude they like and with whom they feel comfortable. Still others use different criteria. The choice is entirely ours. We are free agents and may be coached by anyone who agrees to be our sponsor.

After we secure a sponsor, we can trade him if

necessary, but not merely because he asks us to perform uncomfortable exercises. In fact, guiding uncomfortable rookies through challenging, potentially overwhelming tasks and decisions is one of the sponsor's main functions. These exercises prepare us for the unexpected challenges that will be thrown at us, in one form or another, throughout the course of our lives.

Our sponsor is our confidant. Whatever we say or do our sponsor keeps in strict confidence. When we reveal our darkest secrets to our sponsor, we are usually amazed to find that he isn't shocked. This is important because all addicts (and non-addicts, too) have done things of which we're ashamed and which we would prefer not to discuss. The fact that we can trust our sponsor with our secrets allows us to grow. By revealing our shameful acts, we feel relief and a new freedom. In knowing we are working to change ourselves, we are unlikely to commit such acts in the future. And in knowing that we have a coach behind us, we are likely to succeed.

As we progress through recovery, our sponsor provides us with the benefit of his experience and, anonymously, that of other addicts he knows. But we must provide the hustle. A guide cannot train or climb the mountain for the climber. Don't worry though, our sponsor won't ask us to do anything more than we can handle. One of the first things he's likely to ask us to do is talk about our relationship with alcohol and other drugs.

POWERLESSNESS

*"I'm throwing twice as hard as I used to,
but the ball isn't going as fast."*

➤ Lefty Gomez,
National Baseball Hall of Fame pitcher

Meet Jim Racquet. Jim is an average tennis professional. Although Jim's recent play has been poor, he somehow finds himself playing in the finals at Wimbledon. It will be, as far as he knows, the only time he will have this amazing opportunity. Jim is familiar with his opponent, Buzz. Jim has played Buzz in the past, so he thinks he knows Buzz's style of play. Years ago, Jim beat Buzz by serving into the far corner. Jim likes that serve, and he thinks it fits his game.

Jim begins the match, intent on using the same corner serve. He executes his plan, and Buzz consistently returns Jim's serves, hitting winners up the line. Something has changed. Jim loses his service games and is quickly down a set.

In the next set, our friend employs the same strategy as in the first. He serves to the corner, and Buzz makes him look like a fool. Observers wonder what's wrong with Jim. He loses another set. So far,

Jim's insistence on using that serve has created the ugly situation in which he now finds himself. He has lost control of the biggest match of his life, and his chance to win is seriously threatened.

What should Jim do? Should he cling to distant memories of beating Buzz with his corner serve, or should he acknowledge the score and adjust his game plan?

Many of us confront the same type of situation when it's time to quit drinking or using. As with Jim's chance to play in the Wimbledon finals, as far as we know, we all have just one shot at life. Taking the first drink or drug when we know our drinking and using (like Jim's corner serve) causes us problems only leads us to lose more points, games, and sets. For many of us, our drinking or using has repeatedly resulted in negative physical, social, legal, and psychological consequences. As a result, we eventually lose our spirit.

■ ■ ■

"Before you can win a game,
you have to not lose it."

➤ Chuck Noll,
Pro Football Hall of Fame coach

When we drink or use, losing the match is merely a matter of time. Our drinking or using prohibits us from making conscious decisions about our life's direction, and because the ability to direct is the ability to manage, we cannot manage our lives. This is not a value judgment. It simply means that addiction is winning.

Rather than correctly viewing our use of alcohol or other drugs as the problem, we deny the truth and identify other factors, people, and circumstances as the primary source of our problems. We then use alcohol and drugs as "medicine" to treat the problems caused by using alcohol and drugs. This causes us more problems and makes the problems we already have more severe. If we fail to recognize it, the addictive cycle will thrive and we will continue going back to that first drink or drug for relief. Once we have recognized addiction as the destructive cycle running our lives, however, we are given a choice. We can either continue getting unnecessarily beaten up by drugs, or we can begin our recovery by acknowledging our situation.

We acknowledge our situation by admitting the truth—we can't win if we continue drinking or using, we don't like who we've become, and our alcohol and other drug consumption (not other people, places, or things) is the root of the problem. *Drinking and using doesn't work, and it never will.* When we start drinking or using, our physical reaction is to have more, a compulsion so strong that we are powerless to control the amount we consume. Admitting powerlessness over alcohol and other drugs is not a weakness; it is a sign of strength and flexibility. Calm acceptance of the truth also shows humility and dignity.

At this point in our lives, if we want to stay in the match, we don't have the luxury of giving up a few more points to see if it might work. Like Jim Racquet, we need to acknowledge the way things are and make a change. The match isn't lost yet. We can still win, but it requires abandoning the addiction game and getting into the flow of a positive way of life.

SPIRITUALITY

"If it had not been for the wind in my face, I wouldn't be able to fly at all."

— Arthur Ashe,
International Tennis Hall of Fame

On a blustery day in 1954, England's Roger Bannister ran a mile to avenge his defeat in a race he was supposed to win, the 1952 Olympic 1500-meter. With only a thousand people looking on, Bannister sought to do what no one thought possible and physicians of the day had warned against—break the four-minute barrier. His only real opponents were himself and the clock.

Bannister's Olympic loss had left him disappointed beyond belief. It also motivated him. "If I had gotten a gold medal, I probably would have retired and never pursued the four-minute barrier," he later recalled.

On the morning of the run, Bannister did his rounds at St. Mary's Hospital in London, where he was an intern, fresh out of medical school. After rounds, he sharpened his track spikes and coated them with graphite. The weather was bad, and he hoped the graphite would repel any buildup of discarded power plant ash that coated running tracks of that era. It certainly didn't seem like a good day to break the world record of 4:01, which had stood for the past nine years.

"It was raining, with high winds, and that adds about four seconds [to your time]. So, you're impelled to do the things you can," Bannister recalled. His coach, Franz Stampf, provided confidence. He thought Bannister could run 3:56—break a decade-old record, not to mention the psychological four-minute barrier, by five seconds, even with the bad weather. Stampf's confidence helped Bannister feel that he could do it. He had to do it. Bannister took the train from the hospital to the Oxford University track.

With two men pacing him, Bannister ran the first

three quarters in 3:00.5. He was behind, but he didn't panic. He kept a steady pace until, with about three hundred yards to go, he took off. The crowd went nuts as Bannister flew through the final turn, crossed the finish line, and collapsed, barely conscious. The crowd was hushed. He was helped to his feet as his time was announced. "Three minutes . . ."

The rest of Bannister's time couldn't be heard over the cheers. It didn't matter. England's new hero had redeemed himself. Within three years, sixteen other runners had run sub-four-minute miles. Eventually, America's Steve Scott alone would run 136 sub-four-minute miles and New Zealand's John Walker, 135. In combination with supreme talent and diligent training, Bannister's effort was powered by an intangible force that allowed him to make commonplace what had seemed impossible.

■ ■ ■

"The greatest accomplishments occur not when you do something for yourself, but when you do something for other people."

➤ Ronnie Lott, Pro Football
Hall of Fame safety and cornerback

In every sport, there is a force with a presence that is distinct from the game itself and from the players' physical abilities. A golfer on a hot streak talks of "finding his rhythm." Baseball sluggers get in "a zone" at the plate. Michael Jordan was described as "unconscious" when he scored sixty-three points against the Boston Celtics in a 1986 playoff game. The force accounts for many of the intangibles that so often determine the difference between winning and losing.

When players flow with the force, they achieve great feats. They let go, trusting in the intangibles. Mind, body, and spirit work in perfect coordination. There seems little, if any, resistance as players and teams "find something extra." In the world of recovery, our belief in a greater force is referred to as spirituality. Like athletes, we benefit when we live in coordination with a greater power. Rather than fighting to control everything, we learn to surrender and simply let things happen, allowing the seemingly impossible to become reality.

If we accept as true the proposition that we *are* as we *do*, our continued drinking and using tells us that we value alcohol and drugs more than we value our families, friends, jobs, homes, and more. To value booze and dope more than family and friends is insane. After all, sane people wouldn't drink if booze compromised the good things in their lives. As baffling as it seems, we often don't even realize that there is an alternative.

Going from the insanity of addiction to the sanity of sobriety is a great feat. It requires the power of a force greater than our own. When we let go of our will, we allow the greater force to coordinate body, mind, and spirit to help us stop drinking and using other drugs. The force also clears our vision. It allows us to see accurately the way we have been living and gain the ability to choose the valuable things in life over drinking and using. We find ourselves in our own *zone* where humbly doing the right things seems effortless, and the points we score add up to happiness.

A willingness to utilize a greater power to help us live without alcohol and other drugs is part of our contract. We stop drinking and drugging, commit to doing our best, and have faith that a greater force will show us the path to happiness. As we experience positive results, our faith quickly becomes a genuine belief.

The fact that a greater force has helped millions of people stop drinking and using other drugs should be enough proof for us to have faith that it can work for us, too. When it does, we can continue utilizing the greater power for other purposes, including helping our team win. We, our families, friends, fellows, and the world will all win. If we're still skeptical about whether we can live happily without alcohol and other drugs, it helps to think of ourselves as post-Bannister runners who want to run sub-four-minute miles. We find out how others did it and follow their example.

It is important to note that spirituality does not necessarily mean organized religion, although religion, God, the Buddha, Allah, or any other deity or spiritual force may contribute to, or define, an individual's spirituality. Spirituality is to religion what freestyle snowboarding is to the slalom. Spirituality allows for improvisation and individuality, while most religions have more defined standards that apply equally to all followers. Both spirituality and religion acknowledge the existence of and encourage interaction with a force that has power greater than individual human beings possess.

TEAM PLAY

"The secret of winning football games is working more as a team, less as individuals. I play not my 11 best, but my best 11."

— Knute Rockne,
College Football Hall of Fame coach

David Robinson ("The Admiral") was an instant sensation when he entered the NBA (National Basketball

Association) in 1990. His game was amazing. At 7'1", he could score, pass, run the floor, and play defense. He once blocked twelve shots in a single game. In another, he scored seventy-one points. By 1995, Robinson had earned Rookie of the Year, Defensive MVP (Most Valuable Player), and league MVP honors. He was a legitimate superstar. Still, his team, the San Antonio Spurs, hadn't won a title.

As the Spurs' leader, Robinson held himself accountable. He was determined to bring a championship to his team, his fans, and his city. But how? Did he need to do more? An individual player could hardly do more than Robinson had. He decided that in order for the team to excel, he needed to do less. When the Spurs brought in Tim Duncan, another man with incredible talent, Robinson humbly relinquished the spotlight.

Rather than doing it all, Robinson used his experience and diverse game skills to play whatever role his team needed in order to win. As a result, his individual stats went down but the Spurs won as never before. By the time Robinson decided to retire, San Antonio had won two world championships. The Admiral's commitment to team play changed him from an individual star player into what he and his team will always be—champions.

Star players typically have a lot of self-confidence. This is understandable. Exaggerated self-confidence, even cockiness, is sometimes necessary to do what they do. Unfortunately, a star's extreme confidence in his athletic ability sometimes becomes extreme confidence in his persona. He becomes bigger than his team and the sport to which he owes everything. His ego causes him to lose perspective of his place in the greater scheme of things.

If it weren't for nature, a star could play well indefinitely and never be forced to outgrow or confront his limited perspective. However, some stars get injured and every star slows down with age. If an aging star is to stay in the game, he must adapt.

How does he begin? Like David Robinson, he becomes willing to accept the fact that he is merely one part of something larger and more important—his team.

A team of committed, selfless players produces results that exceed the sum of each player's individual effort. Its power is one large force with fewer exposed weaknesses that is too much for any individual to stop. Anyone who has played or watched sports knows this truth. Really, it's the beauty of the game. In baseball, is anything better than a come-from-behind rally to win in the ninth?

■ ■ ■

*"Ask not what your teammates
can do for you. Ask what you can
do for your teammates."*

➥ Earvin "Magic" Johnson,
Basketball Hall of Fame

The team concept is valuable to addicts as well. It is immaterial whether an addict is a "star" type while drinking or drugging. Every active addict is selfish, similar to a self-absorbed player. Each puts his own interests before his team's interests. Addicts will go to any length to feel better, even forsaking the good of family and friends.

Then at some point our lives come apart, and we are challenged to confront and outgrow our limited perspective. Living with things as they exist becomes unbearable. This is called "hitting a bottom." When we hit a bottom, we can stubbornly take it to the end as lonely individuals or we can change; we can make our team better by disavowing our unreasonably selfish desires. Our recovery contract requires our commitment to team play.

When we do what is good for our team, we experience positive momentum. We don't fear disaster because we're moving with a unified force that is less exposed. Our moments of weakness will be covered by teammates who "have our back," and in turn, we will provide strength for others when we can.

The satisfaction we receive from contributing to our team's success makes us want to stay sober. The ball starts bouncing our way, and we experience victory after victory. We become optimistic and confident that good things are coming. Like David Robinson, we become champions and have people we love with whom to share our new lives. As we'll see, our team contribution and the satisfaction we receive are proportional to the effort we invest in our fitness.

TRAINING AND CONDITIONING

"Nothing good comes in life or athletics unless a lot of hard work has preceded the effort. Only temporary success is achieved by taking shortcuts."

— Roger Staubach,
Pro Football Hall of Fame quarterback

In 1940, an African American woman named Wilma Rudolph was born prematurely in Tennessee. She was the seventeenth of nineteen children. As a kid, Rudolph contracted pneumonia, scarlet fever, and polio, the same disease that had forced President Roosevelt into a wheelchair. Everything was working against her. She was so sick that her only dream was simply to be healthy.

Despite the fact that African Americans at that time didn't have access to the best doctors or hospitals,

Rudolph survived. Still, there was lasting damage. Her ailments had partially deformed her left leg.

At first, Rudolph needed leg braces in order to walk. To ease her pain, her family massaged her legs. They regularly took her to physical therapy where she worked hard. At age nine, she surprised everyone by walking without braces. At eleven, she was playing hoops for her high school team. As she became stronger, her game improved. She set the Tennessee state record for most points in a high school game. Of all things, it was her speed that made her virtually unstoppable.

With the guidance and encouragement of Ed Temple, Tennessee State University's track coach, Rudolph took her speed from the basketball court to the track. She won every high school race she entered. At age sixteen, she won a bronze medal at the 1956 Melbourne Olympics. She kept training. In 1960, while attending Tennessee State, Rudolph set the world record for the 200-meter dash. She kept training. At the 1960 Rome Olympics, she won gold in the 100- and 200-meter dashes and the 4x100-meter relay, becoming the first American woman to win three gold medals in one Olympics and setting world records in all three events. The sick kid from Tennessee was the fastest woman on earth, a superstar who was adored around the world.

People from virtually every country flocked to see Rudolph in person. Fortunately, fame didn't go to her head. For the rest of her life, she humbly used her notoriety to promote positive social change, including racial integration, youth participation in athletics, and a relationship of goodwill between the United States and West Africa. From childhood to death, this graceful, kind, generous woman trained hard and accepted help from others to make herself healthy and strong, and to make the world a better place.

Like polio and other chronic, progressive diseases, addiction is a relentless opponent. To beat it, we must get in shape. Unlike athletes, addicts don't strive to lift more or run faster. We strive to live by the truth, flow with a greater force, and be of service to others. Still, the advantages gained from good conditioning are similar for athletes and addicts alike.

■ ■ ■

"A champion is someone who is bending over to exhaustion when no one else is watching."

➤ Mia Hamm, Olympic gold medalist and two-time FIFA Women's World Cup soccer champion

Just as an athlete's quality of play improves with greater fitness, so does an addict's quality of life. The maxims "you get out what you put in" and "no pain, no gain" equally apply to athletes and addicts in recovery. Training creates strength, flexibility, balance, and greater endurance.

As addicts, we have a training program that consists of simple, yet crucial exercises that we need to perform thoroughly. First, we honestly look at ourselves and find the parts of our game that do and don't work within our team framework. We then gain strength from a greater force and change our lives by accentuating the parts that work while eliminating the parts that don't. Finally, we drop the weight of our past and build the muscle to move forward by making up for the harm we've caused.

We don't rush through our training exercises. Proper conditioning comes when we work through a progression of steps, one at a time. It requires time, consistency, and determination. No one gets in shape overnight, but positive results will come quickly and continue as long as we provide consistent effort and patience. We begin training by looking at our past, an exercise athletes and sports fans know as viewing game film.

GAME FILM

*"The man who complains
about the way the ball bounces is
likely the one who dropped it."*

— Lou Holtz,
champion college football coach

College football has a long, rich history in America. Each season brings a new opportunity for teams that may have suffered the year before. Throughout the years, there have been some amazing comeback stories, football programs that changed from disgraceful to top-notch, seemingly overnight. Stanford was 1–7–1 in 1939 and 10–0 in 1940. Northwestern had twenty-three straight losing seasons, including a thirty-four-game losing streak, before winning the Big Ten Conference in 1995.

Behind every turnaround is a hidden story, a story of hard work, dedication, and faith. Recently, there have been impressive changes at Boise State and Rutgers Universities. The Pacific-10 Conference (Pac-10) has seen the Oregon Ducks rise from obscurity. It has also seen the awakening of the University of California (Cal) Golden Bears, who now annually challenge the mighty University of Southern California Trojans.

In 2001, the Golden Bears had won just thirteen games in the previous four years. They were easily the worst team in the Pac-10 and one of the worst teams in the country. Although they had talent, the athletes were beaten down. They had stopped performing in the classroom, at practice, and on game day. If the program was going to survive, something dramatic had to be done. The Golden Bears hired a young, new head coach named Jeff Tedford. As a former standout quarterback, Tedford came with an excellent reputation for developing and relating to players.

"I believe Jeff's one of the finest minds in all of football," said NFL quarterback Trent Dilfer. "He's a great leader and a great teacher. He has very high expectations for himself and the people around him. And he will work tirelessly to meet those expectations."

Coach Tedford's tireless effort was evident as soon as he took over at Cal. He and his staff worked day and night, studying game film. They put in the time and effort necessary to evaluate why the team wasn't successful and what was required to prepare for and play the following week as well as possible. The coach slept in his stadium office many nights each week, every week of the season. "It's my responsibility to make sure my players have the answers to the test," he said.

Coach Tedford's approach paid off; his devotion to the team inspired his players to dedicate themselves to reaching their full potential, Tedford's measure of success. In his system, winning, as such, is not the objective. Rather, it is the natural by-product of a progression of positive elements that build on one another, ultimately resulting in success. The progression looks like this: 100 percent Desire, which gives rise to Hard Work, which gives rise to Results, which give rise to Confidence, which leads to Success.

In 2002, Tedford's first season, the Golden Bears went from 1–11 to 7–5, one of the greatest one-year turnarounds in history. Since then, the team has been to four straight bowl games, tied in 2006 for its conference championship, and has been nationally ranked the past five years.

Now, imagine you are in Coach Tedford's situation. You are the head coach of a team that has suffered several painful seasons in a row. Your program is out of control. It has lost the respect of people whose opinion you value. Although no one ever intended to let things slip this way, one thing is certain—your team as it presently exists cannot be successful. Your recent record proves it. You need a different approach.

What changes should you make to build a successful program? First, you need to determine why you have been unsuccessful. In sports, this determination requires an honest evaluation of your game film. In recovery, we conduct a similar type of assessment known as "taking inventory."

■ ■ ■

"It's not whether you get knocked down, it's whether you get up."

➤ Vince Lombardi,
Pro Football Hall of Fame coach

We take inventory by watching our personal game film, replaying events in our memories in order to determine where our lives went astray. By taking inventory, we come to realize that bad luck, such as a genetic predisposition for addiction, does not account for all the damage we have caused to ourselves and to others. There is more. We find it by working backward, first identifying the losses, then determining the causes.

Our losses are the events that have produced our resentments. Resentments make us unhappy because they produce and reinforce a negative outlook. We identify the people, places, and things we resent, then look at the film again, honestly accounting for our own decisions, words, behaviors, or instincts that may have contributed to the situation in any way. In other words, we find our shortcomings that have caused our own unhappiness. These shortcomings are often referred to in recovery as "defects of character."

Finding the things we do that make us unhappy and understanding the reason we do them is essential if we are to rebuild our lives on a strong foundation. The process of evaluating the things in our lives that are valuable and those that aren't gives us a game plan for keeping the good, eliminating the bad, and changing the rest, either by modification or acquisition. After that, success is merely a matter of executing the plan while maintaining a positive state of mind.

In college football, if a team needs a hard-hitting safety, it may be able to recruit one from high school, convert a linebacker or cornerback, or sign a junior college transfer. In recovery, we almost always need confidence and self-esteem. Depending on our situation, we can acquire confidence and self-esteem by working to eliminate our nonvirtuous behavior, continuing the virtuous actions that presently make us feel good about ourselves, adding positive activities, or doing differently some of the things we have always done. We can remain positive by looking for something we're doing right.

This process requires hustle, which, as in Coach Tedford's system, requires 100 percent desire. A half-hearted inventory will yield limited results that may leave us feeling that our efforts didn't work. Our failure to put in the effort required to identify *all* of our character defects is a common cause of many of our relapses into the hell of alcohol and other drug abuse. We check ourselves by looking in the mirror and asking, "Am I giving the right effort?"

To switch sports, a situation in baseball provides a good illustration of the type of effort required when conducting an inventory. It may help if we think of ourselves as a batter trying to get to first base when our team is down by two runs with no one on in the ninth inning. A homer with one swing won't do it. We must get on base. There can be no lapse in concentration, no jogging up the line. Now is the time to dig deep and come forward with everything we have.

BECOMING COACHABLE

*"Practice without improvement
is meaningless."*

— Chuck Knox,
football coaching great

Tiger Woods may have a rival when it comes to dominating the world of professional golf. She is Sweden's Annika Sorenstam, one of the greatest athletes, male or female, in history. This World Golf Hall of Fame member didn't become the first non-American to win the NCAA (National Collegiate Athletic Association) championship as a freshman simply because she has good athletic genes. She hasn't earned more prize money than any woman in history because she's lucky or because she's had a few good days. Instead, Sorenstam's success can be traced back to a bit of advice her father gave her when she was just a girl.

It was a cold, rainy day in Stockholm. Sorenstam called her father, Tom, and asked to be picked up early from the local golf practice range. He came for her. They drove away, past the other kids who were still practicing.

"He didn't say anything when he picked me up,"

Sorenstam said. "But when we drove away, he said, 'I just want you to know there are no shortcuts to success.' I knew what he meant. To get better, you have to practice. Just by saying that, it hurt me that I went home. Because I wanted to be good. And I knew he was right."

From that point on, Sorenstam's athletic career would be characterized by listening to others in order to improve herself and her game. Being coachable had always been important, but it became necessary when she started playing against professionals. As a pro, she did not find instant success.

Sorenstam twice failed to qualify for the LPGA (Ladies Professional Golf Association) Tour, but failure didn't stop her. She played the European tour and developed thorough, yet balanced, practice, training, and study habits. She was no longer the shy girl who intentionally missed putts so that she wouldn't have to give an acceptance speech. She was always pushing herself to become better. Her remarkable play would soon make the golf world—the *entire* golf world—sit up and take notice.

With the help of her longtime coach, Henri Reis, Sorenstam won the U.S. Women's Open back-to-back her first two years on the LPGA tour. But her game still needed work. She needed to become stronger in order to hit the ball farther. So, she hired trainer

Kai Fusser and implemented a five-days-per-week workout regimen. Within three years, Sorenstam went from twenty-sixth in driving distance to first. Her improved distance led her to five Player of the Year awards. It also led to perhaps her biggest honor and her biggest challenge, competing professionally with men.

In 2003, Sorenstam accepted an invitation to play in the men's PGA (Professional Golfers Association) Colonial Open. No woman had played in a PGA event since 1945. Sorenstam brought Reis and Fusser with her. She endured intense media scrutiny and chauvinistic comments, such as male golfing standout Vijay Singh's famous, "I hope she misses the cut." Sorenstam did miss the cut, but she played well, showing poise, humility, and dignity. In doing so, she broke barriers and inspired a generation.

Thanks to Sorenstam, people around the world have seen that anything is possible when we become coachable—learning from the right people and putting in the required effort. To honor the people who have helped her and to teach younger golfers, she founded a golf academy and resort. Reis is the head instructor, and Fusser leads the fitness training. Academy students receive excellent coaching on how to shoot lower scores, coaching captured in Sorenstam's book, *Golf Annika's Way*.

■ ■ ■

*"No excuse in the world
counts for squat."*

➤ Mark Schubert,
Olympic swimming coach

In golf, if players don't count every stroke, they really aren't playing golf. Rather than working on their game to improve their score, some golfers write down a fictional number on their scorecard that represents what they want their score to be. Others bypass the truth by claiming that everyone else cheats, mulligans (do-overs) don't count, the course wasn't fair, and many other excuses. Consequently, they cheat themselves, and the problems with their game remain unchanged.

Golf instructors help players improve their game by quickly identifying problems and making effective suggestions. With an instructor's help, practice, and learning the game, a golfer can legitimately earn lower scores. Soon enough, the player won't be ashamed of his score or feel the need to make excuses.

Addicts have just as many excuses for their past actions as golfers have for a bad round. However, with our sponsor's assistance, we can see our shortcomings accurately and the harm we have caused.

We can determine why we acted the way we did. And most important, we can begin living a life that does not leave us ashamed and consistently disappointed. Bouncing ideas off someone else in order to gain an accurate assessment is effective because it is more difficult to kid others than it is to kid ourselves. Accuracy (reality) is important because addicts frequently live in a dangerous world of fantasy when left alone, creating a fictional score that no one recognizes.

Our fantasies are unrealistic, self-serving expectations that invariably frustrate us when they don't materialize. We rarely search for the role we played in our own disappointments. Instead, we develop new expectations based on a different fantasy of the way things should be or are going to be. Thus, we set ourselves up for further disappointment by ignoring the need to adjust our thinking to "what is."

While it is sometimes difficult, admitting the truth about our thoughts and behavior to someone and something other than ourselves is important. It helps minimize our frustration because it keeps our expectations in check with reality. It also reminds us of our limited, yet important, place in the larger world and helps define achievable goals. We learn what we need to work on in order to improve our lives.

Our recovery program, like most everything in life, is more fun when we do it well. In order to improve, thoroughly assessing our game film and conferring with our coach are essential steps. Once we have accurately identified all of our character weaknesses, we can then find the power to eliminate them and take the next step toward living well.

THE POWER TO CHANGE

*"I'm trying to do the best I can.
I'm not concerned about tomorrow,
but with what goes on today."*

➤ Mark Spitz,
nine-time Olympic gold medal swimmer

In 1966, Nolan Ryan, a nineteen-year-old country boy from Texas, was called up to throw fire for the New York Mets. He hadn't gone to college and hadn't spent much time in the minors, but Ryan's fastball (it came to be known as the "Express") was unlike anything baseball had ever seen. It frequently topped a hundred miles per hour, a record (at the time) in *Guinness World Records*. But throwing a ball hard and being a good pitcher are often two different things.

Flamethrowers like Ryan often don't last because they have problems controlling the ball's location. When he was young, Ryan was no exception. In high school, he broke one batter's arm with a wild pitch and broke the next batter's helmet. The third batter, frightened solid, struck out on three pitches. In the Major Leagues, even the often cocky superstar Reggie Jackson admitted that Ryan frightened him. Ryan's wildness didn't last long, though.

When he arrived in the majors, Ryan worked hard on his delivery, which resulted in more consistent accuracy. He trained hard with his conditioning coaches and took advice from fellow pitchers, such as Tom Seaver, and pitching coaches Tom Morgan and Tom House. Over time, Ryan's diligent, consistent effort produced unequalled success. Before retiring, Ryan played in a record twenty-seven Major League seasons.

"My ability to throw the baseball was a gift," Ryan said during his National Baseball Hall of Fame induction speech. "It was a God-given gift. And I am truly appreciative of that gift. It took me a while to figure that out . . . and when I finally did, I dedicated myself to be the best pitcher I could possibly be."

On his way to 324 Major League victories, Nolan Ryan threw seven no-hitters. Seven! Almost as impressive are his twelve one-hitters. Ryan is the only person to strike out the side on nine pitches in both leagues. Although many consider him to be the greatest pitcher of all time, Ryan never threw a perfect game. Still, his dedication to perfection helped him accumulate a staggering number of near-perfect games.

When Ryan lost a perfect game or a no-hitter, he never lost his focus. In fact, he pitched the rest of the game with an even more intense effort to be perfect. Ryan's record proves the value of continuing to reach for perfection when we haven't been perfect in the past. This is the formula for doing our best, for reaching our potential.

■ ■ ■

"I can't concentrate on golf or bowling. I could concentrate in the ring because someone was trying to kill me. Those bowling pins aren't going to hurt me."

➤ Carmen Basilio, boxing champion

The world's best pitchers throw in thousands of Major League games each year, often without even one of them throwing a single perfect game. Life, having more variables than baseball, makes perfection even more difficult to achieve. In sports and in life, therefore, while our effort may be perfect, we can generally expect imperfect results.

Although we can't expect to be perfect in every way at all times, we *can* be perfect at certain things for limited times. In sports, for instance, goalkeepers frequently achieve shutouts in individual games. *In recovery, we must be perfect by never drinking alcohol or taking other drugs.* It's true that recovery is much more than not drinking, but this is one goal where perfection is not only possible but essential. Our lives depend on it. We achieve this perfect sobriety record by repeatedly avoiding alcohol and other drugs for a limited time—one day. One day at a time, many millions of recovering addicts lead great lives.

As for our efforts to correct our other misplaced instincts and shortcomings, we aspire to perfection but rarely, if ever, achieve it.

The previous sections helped us identify our shortcomings that cause our unhappiness. It makes sense that if we remove these deficiencies, we will become happier. So, in this exercise, we work to eliminate them. Our goal is a balanced state of mind where our expectations are based on our needs rather than our wants. When we achieve this balance, reality can meet our expectations and we'll suffer less disappointment. When we don't get what we think we want, our instinctive reaction will no longer be drinking or behaving shamefully, but acting virtuously by recognizing that we have what we need—sobriety and a desire to gradually improve ourselves—and can help others so that they do as well.

■ ■ ■

"Winning is habit.
Unfortunately, so is losing."

➡ Vince Lombardi,
Pro Football Hall of Fame coach

We find balance by expending energy, previously devoted to excess, to areas where we are deficient. For instance, the act of looking out for others' interests instead of our own is an effective way to transform self-pity into self-esteem. The perception that we don't have enough disappears, allowing us to feel contented.

Like Nolan Ryan, we work every day to achieve perfect balance. When we don't feel up to a particular task, we repeatedly find the extra strength we need by asking for assistance from our sponsor or others in recovery, and by using the same force that helped us stop drinking and using when we couldn't do so by ourselves. Our part is providing the willingness and the footwork.

We will not be perfect, but we can only live to our potential if we strive for perfection. Eventually, balance through moderation becomes habit.

As we'll see in the next section, maintaining balanced instincts and feeling contented with less is easier when we have a sufficient amount of humility.

HUMILITY TRAINING

*"A part of control is learning to
correct your weaknesses."*

➤ Babe Ruth, National Baseball
Hall of Fame slugger and pitcher

Hockey players fight. It's part of the game. In a 1969 exhibition game between the Boston Bruins and the St. Louis Blues, Bruin Ted Green, a player with the reputation of being an "enforcer," swung his stick and hit St. Louis' Wayne Maki on the head. Maki responded by spearing Green in the head with his stick, which fractured Green's skull and required the surgical insertion of a metal plate in his head. Green was out the entire season, and Maki was tried criminally for assault. This example is extreme, but even small violations can bring serious consequences.

When a hockey player is penalized for fighting or rough play, he is forced off the ice and his teammates must play with one player short of a full team. It's called a "power play," and it handicaps the penalized team. Most players who enjoy fighting don't do it at crucial moments in a game. They don't want to risk being thrown in the penalty box, placing the game's outcome in jeopardy.

On the other hand, a purely reactionary player who can't control himself will fight regardless of the circumstances in the game. The fighter is proud. He'll high-stick, cross-check, and rough up other players whenever it suits him. He is thrown into the box repeatedly, forcing his team to play shorthanded. His impulsive behavior causes his team to lose.

Although an impulsive fighter may be well liked and even respected, the team can't continue risking important games by putting him on the ice. Sooner or later, he gets benched or booted from the team. This man's problem is obvious to everyone except, perhaps, himself. An addict often finds himself in a similar situation.

■ ■ ■

> *"A life is not important, except*
> *in the impact it has on other lives."*
>
> ➤ Jackie Robinson, National Baseball
> Hall of Fame infielder-outfielder

Addicts are proud people. Our instincts tell us that we should be able to do what we want, when we want, but our self-serving verbal and physical behavior compromises our ability to live in harmony with ourselves, our loved ones, and society in general.

One essential antidote to our misguided instincts is humility. Humility is the opposite of pride. Where pride is the weakness that blinds us to the truth, humility is the strength that allows vision. Pride makes us rigid, stubborn, and susceptible to injury, which is one reason that addicts tend to be overly sensitive and easily hurt by otherwise innocuous incidents.

Humility, on the other hand, results in and is the result of flexibility, balance, and the assuredness to give of ourselves, when possible. Humility comes to us when we see that going through life "our way" causes damage. When we see that our best thinking got us where we are today, we become willing to ask for help and accept it when it comes. Our egos shrink and, with help, we can acknowledge and change the truth about ourselves.

The truth is not an assessment involving good and bad, but simply a statement of what is. Good players don't whine to the refs about a bad call when the truth is that they're playing poorly. When those of us in recovery humbly accept the truth about ourselves, we have little to complain about and we don't react out of fear. We aren't putting up a front, so we don't feel the need to defend ourselves. This is the freedom often referred to in recovery as "relief from the bondage of self."

When we humbly admit the truth, we begin to improve ourselves. And when we allow others to help us improve ourselves, they experience an increased sense of purpose. In this way, our humility makes the world a better place for them as well. No one is the center of the world, and other people's happiness is just as important as our own. Had Green and Maki kept this in mind, the Bruins and Blues may have won a few more games in 1969. In the next section, we'll discuss how humility helps us tap into an additional source of happiness—cleaning up our past.

SQUARING UP THE PAST: MAKING AMENDS

"When you make a mistake, there are only three things you should ever do about it: 1. admit it; 2. learn from it; and 3. don't repeat it."

➤ Paul "Bear" Bryant,
College Football Hall of Fame coach

Before we enter recovery, when we are practicing addicts reaching new lows, we speak and act in ways that damage our teams. We hurt our family, friends, neighbors, and employers, among others. In doing so, we also impair our ability to live at peace with ourselves. If we fail to acknowledge and learn from our mistakes, like a hitter in a slump, we go to the plate the next time thinking of our past failures. The result is reduced self-esteem and confidence.

When we lack confidence, we live in fear and become anxious.

If we want to feel confident and continue playing for our team, we need to acknowledge our past misdeeds and make amends for them. We may not relish the thought of doing it, but it's a small price to pay for the opportunity to be trusted again and to play with confidence.

The amends exercises require the most courage to carry out, and consequently, they are the exercises that do the most good. The process is similar to what a football player might experience: he loses weight, builds muscle, and gains confidence during two-a-day drills before the season starts. These exercises build a solid foundation of fitness that is essential for long-term recovery. Completing the process gives us the following benefits:

- It clears the air. If in the future we deal with a person we've harmed, our relationship won't be determined by the past. If we have no future together, we can part ways knowing where we stand.
- It frees up the space formerly filled with guilt and shame. We can now occupy that space with our vision of, and plan for executing, a more positive way of thinking and acting.

- It requires that we take responsibility for our actions, building the confidence and self-esteem necessary to grow.
- It reminds us of our poor behavior and the harm it caused, creating a deterrent to slipping back into our formerly self-absorbed lifestyle.

In time, blown relationships heal, and we enter new relationships with the confidence of a .340-hitter coming to the plate. We'll still make outs because that's the nature of the game, but we will not harm people in the same way that A-listed our demotion to the minors.

THE SEARCH

"I hated every minute of training, but I said, 'Don't quit. Suffer now and live the rest of your life as a champion.'"

➤ Muhammad Ali, three-time world heavyweight boxing champion

Compton, California, is a rough place to grow up. Gangs, drugs, and violence rule the streets. Poverty and limited opportunity also make it a very difficult place from which to break free. That's part of the reason the story of Serena Williams and her big sister Venus is so remarkable. What's also amazing is that they left Compton by playing tennis, a primarily Caucasian-dominated sport of affluence.

There have been other African American tennis greats, such as Althea Gibson, Arthur Ashe, and Jeff Blake, but that's only a few people in a sport that dates back to eleventh-century French monks. Under their father's tutelage, Serena and Venus not only broke free of Compton, their journey took them to the top of the tennis world. They have overcome both personal and professional challenges along the way. This is especially true of Serena, whose pro career has been plagued by a chronic injury.

Tennis players' careers tend to be measured by how the athletes do in Grand Slam events: Wimbledon, the French Open, the U.S. Open, and the Australian Open. In 1995, at age fourteen, Serena turned pro and focused on the difficult task of winning a Grand Slam title. In 2003, just eight years after turning pro, Serena won all four Grand Slam titles in a single year. Amazingly, she defeated her sister in the finals each time. When the "Serena Slam" was complete, the young woman from Compton was the world's number one tennis player.

Serena didn't have much time to enjoy her success. In a few months, she had surgery to repair a partial tear in the quadriceps tendon of her left knee. Then, things got worse. The rock of the Williams family, Serena and Venus's beloved older sister Yetunde, was driving down the street in Compton when she was gunned down by a gang member who was trying to hit a different passenger in the car. The family was devastated, but Serena was determined to continue playing, using Yetunde's memory as a source of strength.

■ ■ ■

*"You slam the bottom and
either walk away or suck it up
and get through it."*

➤ Gabrielle Reese, volleyball great

Serena rehabbed her knee and enjoyed some success, but the knee kept giving her trouble. She withdrew from tournament play and worked even harder in physical therapy. While away from the game, her ranking fell as low as 139th in the world. Then, she started playing again. When the 2007 Australian Open began, Serena was unseeded, ranked seventy-ninth in the world. It had been four long years since the Serena Slam, but she was ready. She had taken the time and put in the work necessary to heal properly. Yetunde remained her hidden source of strength.

Serena ripped through her matches, one by one,

beating some of the world's greatest players. In the finals, she lost only three games to the world's (then) number one player, Maria Sharapova. Prior to her match with Serena, Sharapova had lost only one set during the entire tournament. Serena Williams was back on top. She graciously dedicated her latest Grand Slam title to Yetunde.

Now, let's consider a hypothetical scenario: Serena's physician, Dr. Rodney Gabriel, while viewing the X ray and MRI of Serena's knee, sees her partially torn tendon. He opens up the knee to repair the tendon. While he has the knee open, he sees something that didn't show up on the film—loose bone chips. What should he do?

Obviously, Dr. Gabriel would remove the chips because they would diminish Serena's strength, hinder her range of motion, and may cause more damage if left behind. As Serena healed and started playing again, she would discover power and flexibility that she'd forgotten she ever had. When she chased down a lob or approached the net, she'd surprise herself with speed only seen in the distant past.

Similar to an athlete's torn tendons and unseen bone chips, an addict's damaged relationships cause weakness and restricted flexibility. They hurt, they're distracting, and they can cause more damage. An exhaustive search for past damage begins to unleash the burdens of our past and sets our minds at ease.

Our initial search almost certainly will reveal additional damage. We should not shy away from these revelations but welcome their discovery as necessary for proper healing.

Eventually, like Serena with her repaired knee, we will be elated with the results. We will begin living again without the negative thoughts and emotions that unknowingly weighed us down and helped cause our undesirable behavior.

THE PREPARATION

*"You hit home runs not by chance,
but by preparation."*

➤ Roger Maris, baseball slugger

Sports references aside, personal relationships are the most important things in life. Addicts recognize this. We are acutely concerned with how we are perceived by others. Further, we often maintain the delusion that we are seen as we see ourselves. The shame and remorse of our past misdeeds gives us the perception that others regard us poorly. This is a significant source of the overwhelming anxiety and low self-esteem we experience.

Anxiety and low self-esteem are the reasons we become defensive and shut people out, secretly fooling ourselves that "what they don't know can't hurt me." We rationalize, claiming we can do without the people our own behavior has alienated. As a result, we alienate more and more people. Our world becomes small and isolated.

Conversely, when we become willing and attempt to repair damaged or broken relationships, we receive a huge return. In taking responsibility for our actions, we're able to forgive ourselves for what we have done, and we gradually gain self-respect. If we are prepared to give our best effort, without offering excuses, we almost have succeeded already.

■ ■ ■

"The will to win is grossly overrated. The will to prepare is far more important."

➤ Bobby Knight,
Basketball Hall of Fame college coach

To gain the courage necessary to overcome our fear of making amends, we reassure ourselves that the benefits will outweigh any imagined consequences. We get psyched up, knowing we will not shy away from saying and hearing everything necessary. We have worked too hard to get to this point and stand to benefit too much to give it anything less than our best.

We prepare by getting ready to explain to the

person we wronged the reasons we believe we acted the way we did. This usually involves our powerlessness over our drug of choice and may also involve one or more of our other shortcomings. Next, we prepare to say that we are sorry for what we have done and that we now are willing to repair the damage. We also must be ready to listen to the response. Finally, we must be prepared to follow through on our promises to repair the damage, regardless of how daunting any task may appear.

We may feel hesitant to make amends because we forecast unpleasant responses. However, experience has proven that these imagined responses usually don't materialize. The fact is that no one knows what the response will be, so *presupposing any reaction is a waste of time and energy.*

THE EXECUTION

"Forget your opponents;
always play against par."

➤ Sam Snead,
World Golf Hall of Fame golfer

Players in every sport get nervous before playing in a big game, particularly if it's their first time in that setting. Picture a shortstop in his first Major League game. Just called up from the minors, he stands in the infield, surrounded by players he's only read about or seen on TV. His parents, friends, new manager, the television audience, and thousands of screaming fans are watching. Adding to the pressure are the facts that his team really needs this game and that the ball will find him—it always finds the new guy.

■ ■ ■

"Show me a guy who's afraid to look bad, and I'll show you a guy you can beat every time."

➤ Lou Brock, National Baseball Hall of Fame outfielder and base stealer

Our shortstop can't hear very well because his pounding heart causes his brain to hum like crickets. He feels overwhelmed, but he also knows that he is prepared and has what it takes to play in this league. The batter steps into the box. The pitch. Crack! A shot to the hole. Instinctively, the rookie breaks to his right, backhands a short hop, plants, and throws to first. The umpire calls the runner out on a close play. As the ball is thrown around the horn, our man relaxes. His preparation has paid off. He knows he can do it again.

This is what it's like for an addict making an amend. We take the field when we meet with the person we have harmed. We engage in cordial conversation. Like the rookie shortstop, we're nervous, but regardless of our nerves, we must make the play. Here's how we do it: We state why we need to talk to the person. Next, we admit that we were wrong, apologize, and promise to make good on all of the harm we have caused that person. Then, we follow through.

THE FOLLOW-THROUGH

"I am not concerned with your liking
me or disliking me. . . . All I ask is that
you respect me as a human being."

➤ Jackie Robinson, National Baseball
Hall of Fame infielder-outfielder

After Willie Mays had been in the Major Leagues just a few weeks, he begged his manager to send him back down to the minors. He didn't think he could hit Major League pitching. Most people don't remember that Willie started his batting career by going 1–26, or .039. Of course they don't. Willie became arguably the greatest baseball player of all time. With a twenty-three-year career average of .302 and 660 home runs, he could also run, field, and throw at least as well as anyone in his day. He made up nicely for his poor start.

In general, people don't dwell on the bad times.

In sports and in life, what's more important is what we've done for them lately. If we've done our best and they still remember the bad times, there's probably not much we can do about it.

Experience shows that the persons we have harmed may not even remember the incidents for which we seek to make amends. If they do remember, many recognize the courage required to make amends and meet us halfway. Then again, they may yell a bit. This is okay. Listening to a little yelling probably isn't too much for us to pay, in light of our past behavior.

Remember, our purpose in making amends is to make the situation as good as possible for both parties. If it turns out that a person we have wronged doesn't respond positively, that may be as good as the situation will allow. Whether a reaction is positive or negative, *the value of the amend comes from our honest intent and our effort, not the outcome.*

■ ■ ■

> *"I took a different path, one you might not expect. But along the path, I learned about my life—about life."*
>
> ➤ Jennifer Capriati, tennis champion

So, once we've expressed our intent to a person we have harmed, we follow through on our promises, regardless of how we feel about the situation. When our actions match our words, we walk away feeling both relief and self-respect. We keep in mind that baseball players who have broken a slump sometimes become distracted when they again find themselves in the fickle media's good graces. We cannot allow that to happen to us.

In order to avoid slipping into another slump, we must remain focused on the fundamentals, doing the things in life that make us successful. Part of our follow-through is our continuing effort to cast away character defects and get in the habit of being virtuous, including being honest, grateful, and humble. We always need to keep an honest eye on ourselves and avoid becoming too high or too low when we hear others' opinions about our progress. When we become too low, we may become depressed and lose our motivation to continue improving. When we get too high, we may feel like we have arrived and no further action is necessary on our part. Our reaction to compliments is especially important.

After receiving amends, those we have wronged often tell us that we have changed for the better. They sometimes say that we've improved so much that we seem like a completely different person. We cannot let such comments affect our motivation to continue improving ourselves. While a compliment may be interesting, addicts should keep in mind that it may be the result of incomplete information. They may only be seeing our good sides without knowing everything that is going on inside of us.

The person we have wronged also may have a lower standard of behavior than the one to which we now aspire. Some of the companions we hung-out with during our drinking and using years may validate even our most regressive, selfish behavior by telling us "it wasn't that bad." Joe Paterno, college football's winningest head coach, once said, "Publicity is like poison. It only hurts if you swallow it." We're better off sticking with what we know to be the truth. Other people's opinions, good or bad, don't allow us to sleep well at night. Deep sleep comes from within us, from working to improve ourselves, contributing to our team, and knowing we'll continue to do so.

THE UNATTAINABLE

*"The sterner the discipline,
the greater the devotion."*

➤ Pete Carril,
Basketball Hall of Fame college coach

Overtraining can be dangerous. Athletes must be careful that their zeal for fitness doesn't cause harm and defeat the purpose of being in shape. Likewise, in recovery we must sometimes restrain ourselves from attempting to make an amend because it may cause harm and defeat the purpose of the process. We should exercise the discipline necessary to leave certain people alone. We can't build our own peace of mind at others' expense.

There may also be people to whom we cannot make direct amends because they have died or cannot be located. In such cases, we should confer with our sponsors. So long as we have the desire to make as much reparation as possible, we are usually on the right track. We have laid a solid foundation. We can now work on maintaining our healthy, productive lives on a daily basis.

GAME/RACE DAY

"You get out in front.
You stay out in front."

➤ A.J. Foyt,
champion NASCAR driver

Imagine yourself as a twenty-eight-year-old bio-
medical researcher. When you're away from your
laboratory job, you enjoy riding your mountain bike.
Bicycling is your passion. You consider yourself a
skilled, strong rider, and you dream about racing
bikes for a living, rather than conducting laboratory
research. You ask yourself, "Should I do it? Should I
quit this well-paying job, risk everything, and chase
the irrational dream of extreme sports competition,
racing against more experienced riders who are much
younger than me?" For Marla Streb, the answer was
"yes." She quit her job and hopped on her bike. She
started training and racing, chasing down her dream.

One of many things that makes Streb extraordinary is that she races downhill events in addition to the grueling, long-distance cross-country races. Most mountain bikers are specialists, choosing one type of race or the other. Each type of racing has unique mental and physical requirements. But Streb liked both, she was good at both, so she raced both.

At first, her results were inconsistent. She crashed a lot. Significantly, she responded by getting up and trying again. High-speed crashes are simply part of mountain biking, the price of gaining precious racing experience. Streb also responded by refining her training methods and learning how to take better care of herself on a daily basis. She learned what her body needed before, during, and after a race in order for her to perform her best.

Soon, Streb's results improved. She became more consistent and started winning big races. In 2003 and 2004, she was the U.S. National Downhill Champion and was Single-Speed World Champion twice. Ten years after she turned pro, at age thirty-eight, her career was peaking. Her racing success and have-fun attitude have made Streb an extreme-sports icon. "Enjoy it now before you get eaten by worms and bugs," she likes to say.

Today, Streb uses her notoriety for charitable purposes, promoting the Breast Cancer Fund on behalf of her sponsor, the LUNA Women's Mountain Bike

Team. Streb has also written two books on biking. Both spell out the need to monitor and take care of your body consistently in order to achieve the best possible results.

■ ■ ■

"The secret to winning is constant, consistent management."

➤ Tom Landry,
Pro Football Hall of Fame coach

A competitive mountain biker must be in top condition. If she doesn't maintain excellent fitness, eat right, and pace herself well during a race, she will "bonk." Bonking is exhaustion so severe that the suffering biker believes that continuing to ride is impossible. The pain in her body causes her mind to give up. To say the least, it is an unpleasant experience. Even the most talented and fit athletes bonk if they fail to monitor themselves.

Addicts also risk bonking as sobriety progresses. Our bonks are painful to the spirit and cause us to lose our ability to make good decisions, such as resisting self-interested, destructive behavior. We bonk because we fail to continue doing the things that got us in shape, the same exercises that allowed us to quit drinking and using, and helped make our lives better.

The encouraging thing is that bonking is entirely

avoidable. A mountain biker will not bonk if, every day, she trains consistently and properly, gets enough rest, drinks and eats correctly, and on race day, she does not ride too hard at the start. Similarly, as recovering addicts, we avoid bonking by consistently taking care of our manner of living. Like Streb, we need to exercise, eat right, hydrate properly, rest enough, and pace ourselves throughout the day.

We also maintain our lifestyles by looking at our game film on a daily basis and by making any adjustments necessary. For instance, when we treat someone poorly, we admit we were wrong and apologize right away. Falling into our old bad habits is easy if we don't check them regularly. We also make sure that our motivations are focused on our priorities, rather than on unhealthy distractions. Looking at ourselves truthfully and doing our best on each and every day is the key.

FOCUSING ON TODAY'S GAME

"Somebody will always break your records. It is how you live that counts."

➤ Earl Campbell, Pro Football
Hall of Fame running back

Each day provides a new opportunity to improve. Consider this: In August of 1951, baseball's New York

Giants were down by thirteen and one-half games to the Brooklyn Dodgers. There was only about a month left in the season. Winning the National League pennant appeared impossible, but the Giants had been playing good ball lately. Manager Leo Durocher challenged his players. He conceded that they may not catch the Dodgers in the end, but they should continue playing hard, game by game, just to see how close they could come.

■ ■ ■

"Whatever your goal in life,
be proud of every day you are able
to work in that direction."

➤ Chris Evert, International Tennis
Hall of Fame player

The Giants played as their manager suggested. They ended up tying the Dodgers on the last day of the season, forcing a three-game playoff. In the final inning of the final playoff game, the Giants beat the Dodgers with Bobby Thomson's legendary home run, known as the "Shot Heard 'Round the World." The Giants went on to meet (and lose to) Joe DiMaggio, rookie Mickey Mantle, and the rest of the Yankees in the World Series. Had the Giants paid attention to the overall standings in August, rather than concentrating on each day's game, they surely wouldn't have made it to the World Series.

As much as possible, recovering addicts carry the 1951 Giants' mind-set every day. We live as well as we can and do not worry about what will happen tomorrow or in the future. The end result becomes less important to us when we come to realize that living each day as well as possible is its own reward. Daily inventory and promptly admitting fault are essential exercises that allow us to maintain our healthy lives.

MAINTAINING FUNDAMENTAL FITNESS

*"Hard work made it easy.
That is my secret. That is why I win."*

➤ Nadia Comaneci,
five-time Olympic gold medal gymnast

A golfer uses his putter on every hole, which is the reason that the putter is the most frequently used club in golf. A two-inch putt is worth one stroke, the same as a three-hundred-yard drive. Thus, putting is a golfer's most important skill. When teaching their students to putt, instructors emphasize "the speed and the read." The speed is how hard to hit the ball, and the read is where to aim it. Successful golfers develop and maintain their feel for the correct distance and direction through consistent efforts to improve.

Multiple factors work against a golfer as he works to improve his putting stroke. The golfer himself changes, the weather changes, and every golf course is different. So, even after developing a proficient feel, a golfer must continually practice in order to maintain it.

The same principles that allow a golfer to post a low score through good putting apply to addicts seeking a happy, healthy manner of living. We must learn the correct power and direction for our lives, developing our own feel for life's speed and read. With practice, we find the activities we can do and the amount we should do them in order to live honest, balanced lives. Once we've developed our feel, it takes consistent effort to maintain, keeping an eye on what we're doing and how busy we are. If we let ourselves do the wrong things, try to do too much, or become complacent or neglectful, our lives will move off course, breaking either too fast or not fast enough. When we develop and maintain a good feel for speed and direction, we stand an excellent chance of achieving our potential.

■ ■ ■

"Success is like surfing;
you're doing what you can to stay
on board, but you really aren't
in charge of anything."

➤ Kirk Shelmerdine,
NASCAR crew chief, owner, and driver

An indispensable element for those of us who want to achieve our potential is the continuing development of our soul—our spirit. Notoriety, recognition, and personal gain are no longer the goals, although perhaps pleasant by-products of selfless behavior. To develop our spirituality, we persistently put our wants behind others' needs, trying to make others' lives better. We seek assistance in our quest by tapping into a greater spiritual power, the force described above, for courage and guidance.

When we appeal to a force greater than ourselves, we then can begin to understand our smaller, individual role by simply asking the same force to guide us, showing us what our role is. We will discover our individual roles when we slow down, stop trying to run the show, and take the time to listen, feel, and open our eyes.

As our role becomes clearer, we ask for the power

to carry out our part. Our appeal for direction and strength may not yield easy or immediate results, but good results will come. Maintaining our spirituality is an essential, enjoyable factor that allows us to pass on the formula for our consistently improving lives.

LEADING BY EXAMPLE AND INSTRUCTION

"Leadership must be demonstrated, not announced."

➥ Fran Tarkenton,
Pro Football Hall of Fame quarterback

We often hear reporters ask players about their accomplishments. The more humble players say that some, if not most, of the credit goes to their teammates, coaches, and others who taught them the ropes when they broke in.

Generally, older players teach younger players, but that isn't a rule. In baseball, a veteran catcher may change positions from behind the plate to first base in order to extend his career. A younger first baseman can teach him the skills necessary to master the position. The key element is experience.

Those with more relevant experience and success

help the less experienced become successful by passing along what they have learned. This principle also applies to addicts. Recovery veterans will help us, but we need to reach out to them.

Addicts who have learned to live happily without alcohol and other drugs teach what they have learned to others who are just starting out. In early recovery, if we reach out, we will discover that people who have *been there* genuinely are interested in our happiness. Thus, we may feel we can trust the vets and grant them even more credibility than loved ones, who may view our drinking as something that simply has to stop. The loved ones are correct, but the veteran alcoholics have lived it and know how to get it done.

■ ■ ■

"Friendships born on the field of athletic strife are the real gold of competition. Awards become corroded, friends gather no dust."

◆ Jesse Owens, four-time Olympic gold medalist, track and field

Recovery veterans also benefit from helping others recover. Recovering addicts with some length of sobriety are able to give back to the game. In doing so, we experience the incomparable satisfaction of making the difference between life and death for another person. We are also reminded of the fundamentals that we, in our own lives, may have allowed to slip. Just as a veteran baseball player tells the rookies to run out every ball, he must do so himself. Otherwise, he ain't walkin' the walk. The result is a few extra hits for the old guy, the reason he professed the principle in the first place—because it works.

When everyone on the team is hustling, it's contagious. The team gains a spirit that never says die. If one player isn't hitting, the others pick him up until he's contributing again. Contributing to a winning team is fun, it's healthy, and it's what life is all about. This is especially true in recovery. By working together, we live happy, fulfilling lives without subjecting ourselves to the often fatal consequences that the bottle ensures.

REWRITE THE
RECORD BOOKS

"Don't let anyone steal our dreams."

➤ Michael Jordan,
Basketball Hall of Fame

Many athletes have saved what once appeared to be careers on the downslope. Dennis Eckersley, Chris Mullin, and Andre Agassi are just a few who have made remarkable comebacks. Addicts can do the same if we gain the necessary humility and determination to live truthfully. Happiness is a measure of our contentment with how we're living our lives. In order to become happy, we adopt and stick with a healthy training program. The program I've outlined has proven successful in giving countless recovering addicts satisfaction and contentment in how we live. However, no training program will help us until we acknowledge that, while drinking or using, we're in a two-strike count with a broken bat.

Our training program fuels and guides our continuous effort to improve ourselves within a team context. We are all part of a team that, in turn, is part of a greater force. When the individuals who make up a team acknowledge and move with the force, a winning life seems effortless. In contrast, when acting solely for himself and with disregard for his team and the force, an individual's effort is a frustrating struggle. A team *never* wins solely due to one player's performance, but one player easily can cause a team to lose. Keep in mind that while a good player may bat .310, a good team's winning percentage is over .600.

■ ■ ■

"I've learned it's not always the most talented people who make it, but those who don't give up."

➥ Adam Burt, NHL hockey player

Getting back in the game is a process. The process provides a game plan for gaining the strength, balance, flexibility, and endurance necessary to succeed. Our success becomes defined as helping make others' lives better. When we acknowledge our flawed manner of living, work hard, and ask for help to identify and correct our flaws, past and present, we gain the capacity and desire to contribute selflessly to our team. Throughout the process, we will experience success, and rather than seeking the delusional comfort of distant memories, we will move forward, leaving the desire to drink or use behind.

Like an athlete who is rolling with momentum, scoring points and playing defense, as recovering addicts, we find ourselves in the groove of the force of life. It feels good. We feel that we are where we are supposed to be, doing what we are supposed to be doing. Feeling this way, however, does not come instantly or easily. It requires effort and the humility to accept guidance from our fellows as well as unearthly, supernatural sources.

In soccer, a situation in which the ball is between two opponents, an equal distance from each, is known as a "50/50 ball." A player will either gain possession of the ball or he won't, depending on what happens next. Soccer fundamentals instruct a player who has come upon a 50/50 ball to go after it with everything he has. He cannot make a compromised effort. If a player goes all out, more often than not he will end up with the ball, while the player with less desire suffers the consequences of a half-hearted effort. You or someone you know may be in the same situation.

Happiness through sobriety is available, but to

recover, we must want it. We need to go all out. We can't afford to think about all of the "what ifs" that will paralyze us into fear or the "what could have beens" that will cause depressing remorse. I believe that we can know happiness—*if we truly* want it. So, if *you* need a change, I encourage you to live like your team is playing for the World Cup and go all out. Get some help and *GET THE BALL, BABY!*

■ ■ ■

"Winning is only half of it.
The other half is having fun."

← Bum Phillips, NFL head coach

LEARNING THE LINGO:
PHRASES AND CONCEPTS

"I didn't really say everything I said."

➤ Yogi Berra, National Baseball
Hall of Fame catcher

The terms and phrases of recovery often have different meanings than those found in a dictionary. By interfacing recovery concepts with athletic experience, sports-minded addicts can gain a solid working understanding of recovery.

ADDICTION: A permanent mental and physical condition requiring adjustment to self and style of play

ADDICTION LITERATURE: Playbook; required reading

AMENDS: Catching up; getting square

BOTTOM: Being given your unconditional release; being placed on waivers

CONTROL: Calmly executing a balanced game plan and appropriately adjusting, when necessary

COURAGE: The guts to prepare and execute the elements of a winning game plan

EASY DOES IT: Don't press

EGO: Glory hog; sacrificing team for self and wins for statistics

FAITH: The confidence to punt when behind with four minutes to go, believing your defense will hold

FOUNDATION: Preparation; fitness (practice, stretching, strength training, film, studying playbook); losing the fat

GEOGRAPHIC FIX: Team-hopping with the same deficient game

GRATITUDE: Appreciation for being in the game

HAPPINESS: Performing your best; enjoying the game

HIGHER POWER: The force (momentum) that influences/determines the ebb, flow, and outcome of events in the game of daily life

HUMILITY: Playing to honor your teammates; living truthfully; remembering where you came from; giving credit where it's due; learning your weaknesses; being right sized

IDENTIFY: Situational recognition; substituting someone else's feelings for your own; empathy

INSANITY OF THE DISEASE: Adherence to an ineffective game plan, each time expecting to win despite continuing defeats

IT WORKS IF YOU WORK IT: How you practice is how you'll play; success is 10 percent inspiration and 90 percent perspiration

LETTING GO: Playing only your position; doing your best and accepting the rest

NEWCOMER: Rookie

NINETY MEETINGS IN NINETY DAYS: Spring training

ONE DAY AT A TIME: Play today's game today; fundamentals first

PERSONALITIES: Head fakes

PINK CLOUD: Elation exceeding accomplishment

POWERLESS: Behind in the score when you're playing defense with no time-outs and under two minutes remaining, first and ten

PRAYER: Warming up; stretching; reviewing fundamentals and game plan

PRINCIPLES: The elements of a winning game plan; "why" you play determines "how" you play

PRINCIPLES BEFORE PERSONALITIES: Walking the walk

RECOVERY: Improving yourself to continue playing; maximizing your game

RESENTMENT: Grudge; score to settle; beef

SERENITY: Poise; calm in any circumstance

SERENITY PRAYER: "God, please grant me the

wisdom to recognize a pitch I can hit, the courage to swing when I see it, and serenity to accept
that I will sometimes miss"; look for a pitch you
can drive

SERVICE: Giving back to the team and the game

SHARE: An assist

SLIP: A turnover causing an unnecessary loss

SOBRIETY: Taking care of the ball; holding the lead

SPIRITUAL AWAKENING: A change in one's instinctive approach to playing the game, resulting
from a fundamentally sound perspective

SPIRITUALITY: Tapping into a force; learning the
game; freestyle religion

SPONSOR: Coach; mentor

STEPS OF RECOVERY: Game plan; blueprint

TAKE WHAT YOU NEED: Look for your pitch

TAKING INVENTORY: Viewing game film

TEAM: Family, friends, employer, coworkers,
neighbors

TO THINE SELF BE TRUE: Cover your position; stay
at home

UNMANAGEABLE: Random, directionless, deficient
game plan yielding predictable play and un-
desired results

WISDOM: The insight to develop a winning game
plan

SOURCES AND SUGGESTED READING

BIOGRAPHY AND SPORTS STORIES (IN THE ORDER OF APPEARANCE)

Gale Sayers

Brian's Song. Sony Pictures, 2000.

Pro Football Hall of Fame Official Web site. "Gale Sayers." www.profootballhof.com/hof/member.jsp?player_id=188.

Sayers, Gale, with Al Silverman. *I Am Third: The Inspiration for Brian's Song.* New York: Viking Press, Inc., 1970.

University of Kansas Athletic Web site. "Gale Sayers." www.kusports.com/football/nfl/sayers.html.

Danica Patrick

Associated Press. "Patrick's Shift to Rival Team Begins Friday." Azstarnet.com. November 30, 2006. http://azstarnet.com/sports/158339.

Celebrity-link.com. "D." www.celebrity-link.com/c229/showcelebrity_categoryid-22977.html.

Flies, Peter A. "Articles." All Headline News. November 29, 2006. www.allheadlinenews.com/articles/7005675141 (article no longer available).

Lewandowski, Dave. "News." Indycar.com. July 25, 2006. www.indycar.com/news/story.php?story_id=7176.

McCormick, Steve. "NASCAR Needs Danica Patrick." About.com. http://nascar.about.com/od/otherseries/a/danicapatrick.htm.

The Official Site of Danica Patrick. www.danicaracing.com.

Olson, Jeff. "Danica Patrick Says NASCAR Option Still Open." Speedtv.com. July 14, 2006. www.speedtv.com/articles/auto/indycar/28634.

Patrick, Danica, with Laura Morton. *Danica— Crossing the Line*. New York: Fireside, 2006.

Wikipedia.com. "Danica Patrick." http://en.wikipedia.org/wiki/Danica_Patrick.

Wanda Rutkiewicz

Coffey, Maria. *Where the Mountain Casts Its Shadow: The Dark Side of Extreme Adventure*. New York: St. Martin's Press, 2005.

Curran, Jim. *K2: Triumph and Tragedy*. Boston: Houghton Mifflin Co., 1987.

Jordan, Jennifer. *Savage Summit: The True Stories of the First Five Women Who Climbed K2, the World's Most Feared Mountain*. New York: HarperCollins Publishers, Inc., 2005.

Krakauer, Jon. *Eiger Dreams: Ventures Among Men and Mountains*. New York: Lyons & Burford, 1990.

MountEverest.net. "News." January 31, 2005. www.mounteverest.net.

Reinisch, Gertrude. *Wanda Rutkiewicz: A Caravan of Dreams*. United Kingdom: Careg Ltd., 2000.

Roger Bannister

Bale, John. *Roger Bannister and the Four-Minute Mile: Sports Myth and Sports History*. New York: Taylor & Francis, Inc., 2004, 2005.

Bannister, Roger. *The Four-Minute Mile, Fiftieth-Anniversary Edition*. Guilford: The Lyons Press, 2004.

Clash, James M., "The Adventurer: Four Minutes to Fame," excerpted from Forbes Adventurer Columnist Jim Clash's book, *To the Limits: Pushing Yourself to the Edge—in Adventure and in Business*. (John Wiley & Sons, 2003). Forbes.com. www.forbes.com/lifestyle/collecting/2003/10/21/cz_jc_1021sport.html.

Woolridge, Ian. "How Roger's Historic Run Killed off the Amateur Era." www.DailyMail.co.uk.

May 6, 2004. www.dailymail.co.uk/pages/live/
articles/columnists/columnists.html?in_article_
id=259854&in_page_id=1772&in_author_id=262.

Michael Jordan

NBA.com. "God Disguised as Michael Jordan."
www.nba.com/history/jordan63_moments.html.

David Robinson

AllExperts.com. "David Robinson." http://
en.allexperts.com/e/d/da/david_robinson_
(basketball).htm.
Brown, Jim. "Life is Good in David Robinson's
Neighborhood." *The Sporting News,* July 15, 2005.
Lewis, Gregg, and Deborah Shaw. *Today's Heroes:
David Robinson.* Grand Rapids: Tandem Library,
2002.
NBA.com. "David Robinson." www.nba.com/
history/players/robinson_bio.html.

Wilma Rudolph

Encyclopedia Britannica."Wilma Rudolph." African American World. PBS.org. www.pbs.org/
wnet/aaworld/reference/articles/wilma_
rudolph.html.
Galegroup.com. "Wilma Rudolph." www.galegroup.
com/free_resources/bhm/bio/rudolph_w.htm.

Whitehousekids.gov. "White House Dream Team: Wilma Rudolph." www.whitehouse.gov/kids/dreamteam/wilmarudolph.html.

Women in History Web site. "Wilma Rudolph." www.lkwdpl.org/wihohio/rudo-wil.htm.

Jeff Tedford

Bainum, Brian. "Memorial Mastermind. Coach Jeff Tedford's Attention to Detail and Care for His Players Has Changed the Cal Football Program." Dailycal.org. December 2, 2006. www.dailycal.org/sharticle.php?id=22491.

Biovin, Paola. "Tedford Merits Credit for Rapid Revival." Azcentral.com. September 19, 2006. www.azcentral.com/sports/columns/articles/0919boivin0919.html.

Buchanan, Olin. "Undervalued and Overlooked: The Sleeper Teams." Rivals.com. August 26, 2006. http://collegefootball.rivals.com/content.asp?CID=575730.

CalBears.com. "The Tedford File." http://calbears.cstv.com/sports/m-footbl/mtt/tedford_jeff00.html.

Holterman, Karen. "No. 1 Approach Fuels No. 8 Bears." Berkeley.edu. October 14, 2004. www.berkeley.edu/news/berkeleyan/2004/10/14_tedford.shtml.

Personal interview notes, April 26, 2007.

Annika Sorenstam

Associated Press. "Annika: I'm Not Afraid. Sorenstam Excited about Historic Challenge." GolfDigest.com. December 31, 2003. www.golfdigest.com/newsandtour/index.ssf?/newsandtour/20031213sorenstam.html (article no longer available).

Associated Press. "Before Facing the Field Thursday, Sorenstam Meets the Media." ESPN.com. May 21, 2003. http://sports.espn.go.com/golf/story?id=1556934.

Associated Press. "Daddy Knows Best. Sorenstam Owes Success to Father's Early Lessons." SI.com. October 18, 2003. http://sportsillustrated.cnn.com/2003/golf/10/18/bc.glf.sorenstam.ssucce.ap/index.html.

Associated Press. "It's Annika Again." PGA.com. July 3, 2006. www.pga.com/news/tours/lpga/uswo070306.cfm?rss.

Penick, Harvey, and Bud Shrake. *Harvey Penick's Little Red Book: Lessons and Teachings from a Lifetime of Golf.* New York: Simon & Schuster, 1992.

Sirak, Ron. "Five Days in May: No One Foresaw the Impact of Annika at Colonial. No One Who Saw It Will Forget It." GolfDigest.com. December 19, 2003. www.golfdigest.com/newsandtour/index

.ssf?/newsandtour/20031213sorenstam.html (article no longer available).

Sorenstam, Annika. *Golf Annika's Way: How I Elevated My Game to Be the Best—and How You Can Too.* New York: Penguin Group, 2004.

Wikipedia.com. "Annika Sorenstam." en.wikipedia. org/wiki/Annika_Sorenstam.

Nolan Ryan

BaseballHallofFame.org. "Induction Speeches" (from July 25, 1999 ceremony). www.mingster. org/speech.htm.

BaseballLibrary.com. "Nolan Ryan." www. baseballlibrary.com/baseballlibrary/ballplayers/ R/Ryan_Nolan.stm.

NolanRyanFoundation.org. "Nolan Ryan." www. nolanryanfoundation.org/nolanryan.htm.

Ted Green and Wayne Maki

AllExperts.com. "Wayne Maki." http://en.allexperts. com/e/w/wa/wayne_maki.htm.

Answers.com. "Wayne Maki." www.answers.com/ topic/wayne_maki.

CBC Sports Online. "10 Hockey Violence Lowlights." http://cbc.ca/sports/columns/top10/ hockey_lowlights.html#3.

Wikipedia.org. "Ted Green." http://en.wikipedia.
org/wiki/Ted_Green.

Serena (and Venus) Williams

Associated Press. "Serena Williams to Miss U.S.
Open after Knee Surgery." williamssisters.org.
August 2, 2003. www.venusandserena.
homestead.com/news8203.html.

Cooper, Jeff. "The Origins and Early History of
Tennis." About.com. http://tennis.about.com/
od/history/a/earlyhistory.htm.

Galegroup.com. "Serena Williams." www.galegroup.
com/free_resources/bhm/bio/williams_s.htm.

Kidzworld.com. "Serena Williams." http://
kidzworld.com/article/1294-the-williams-sisters-
venus-and-serena.

Pye, John. "Williams Routs Sharapova, Wins Eighth
Grand Slam Title." williamsisters.org. January
26, 2007. www.venusandserena.homestead.com/
news12607.html.

Wikipedia.org. "Serena Williams." http://
en.wikipedia.org/wiki/serena_williams.

Williams, Venus, and Serena Williams, with Hillary
Beard. *Venus and Serena: Serving from the Hip;
10 Rules for Living, Loving, and Winning.* Boston:
Houghton Mifflin Co., 2005.

Willie Mays

Hano, Arnold. *Willie Mays*. New York: Grosset and Dunlap, 1966.

Mays, Willie, with Lou Sahdi. *Say Hey: The Autobiography of Willie Mays*. New York: Simon and Schuster, 1988.

Marla Streb

Kallal, Mike. "An Interview with Marla Streb: Take a Walk on the Wild Side." Cyclingnews.com. 2003. www.cyclingnews.com/mtb.php?id=riders/2003/interviews/marla_streb03.

Streb, Marla. *Bicycle Magazine's Century Training Program: 100 Days to 100 Miles*. New York: Rodale Inc., 2005. www.rodalestore.com.

Streb, Marla. "Riding into Las Vegas." Mountainzone.com. October 2, 2006. http://mtbike.mountainzone.com/blogs/marla_streb.

New York Giants

A Giants History: The Tale of Two Cities. VHS recording. 3M/Leisure Time Productions/Sportsman Video, 1969.

Thomson, Bobby, with Bill Gutman. *The Giants Win the Pennant! The Giants Win the Pennant!* New York: Citadel, 2001.

University of New Hampshire Pub Pages. "New York Giants: The Land of the Giants." Listen to Russ Hodges call the "Shot Heard 'Round the World." http://pubpages.unh.edu/~mwh4/giants.html.

MISCELLANEOUS SPORTS SOURCES

Armstrong, Lance, with Sally Jenkins. *Every Second Counts*. New York: Random House, 2003.

QUOTATIONS

About.com. "Education Quotations." http://quotations.about.com/cs/inspirationquotes/a/Knowledge1.htm.

Anderson, Peggy, and Rick Gonella. *Great Quotes from Great Sports Heroes*. Franklin Lakes: Career Press, 1997.

Answers.com. "Dictionary-People." www.answers.com.

Anvari.org. "Fortune Cookies." www.anvari.org/fortune/Fortune_Big_F/794.html.

Baseball-Statistics.com. "Hall of Fame Player Index." www.baseball-statistics.com.

Brown, Bruce Eamon. *1001 Motivational Messages and Quotes*. Monterey: Coaches Choice, 2001.

Cybernation.com. "Success Quotation Center." www.cybernation.com/quotationcenter.

DailyCelebrations.com. "Quotations."
www.dailycelebrations.com/quotes.htm.

DecaturSports.com. "A Year's Worth of
Inspirational Quotes." www.dprsports.com/
quotes/quotes_of_the_day.htm.

DeVito, Carlo. *The Ultimate Dictionary of Sports
Quotations*. New York: Facts on File, 2001.

Don'tQuoteMe.com. "Home." www.dontquoteme.
com.

Entplaza.com. "Quotations." www.entplaza.com/
quotations.

Game Plan Media. "Our Playbook." http://
gameplanmedia.com/playbook.

Geocities.com. "Schoonoverb." www.geocities.com/
schoonoverb/index.html.

Green, Lee. *Sportswit*. New York: HarperCollins,
1984.

Liebman, Glenn. *2000 Sports Quips and Quotes*. New
York: Gramercy Books, 1993.

Life Revolution. "Web Log." http://liferevolution.
net/weblog.

Living Destiny. "Quotes for Living."
www.livingdestiny.com/Quotes.htm.

NadiaComaneci.com. "Home."
www.nadiacomaneci.com/index.htm.

Nathan, David H. *Baseball Quotations: The Wisdom
and Wisecracks, Players, Managers, Owners, Umpires,*

Announcers, Writers, and Fans of the Great American Pastime. New York: Ballentine Books, 1991.

Nelson, Kevin. *Baseball's Greatest Quotes*. New York: Simon & Schuster, 1982.

The Official Site of Jackie Robinson. "Quotes." www.jackierobinson.com/about/quotes.html.

The Quotations Page. "Home." www.quotationspage.com.

QuotationsBook.com. "Home." www.quotationsbook.com/quote/39445.

QuoteMountain.com. "Motivational Sports Quotes." www.quotemountain.com/quotes/sports_quotes/motivational_sports_quotes.

Silverman, Al, with Brian Silverman. *Twentieth Century Treasury of Sports*. New York: Viking, Inc., 1992.

Sugar, Bert Randolph. *The Baseball Trivia Book*. New York: Playboy Paperbacks, 1981.

ThinkExist.com. "Home." www.thinkexist.com.

TV.com. "Muhammad Ali Summary." www.tv.com/muhammad-ali/person/34613/summary.html?q=muhammad%20ali&tag=search_results;more;0.

Wikiquote. "Home." http://en.wikiquote.org.

WorldofQuotes.com. "Home." www.worldofquotes.com.

Yogi Berra Official Web Site. "Yogi-isms."
  www.yogiberra.com/yogi-isms.html.

SOBRIETY

A.A. for the Older Alcoholic: Never Too Late. New York:
  Alcoholics Anonymous World Services, Inc.,
  2001.

A.A. for the Woman. New York: Alcoholics
  Anonymous World Services, Inc., 1976.

*Alcoholics Anonymous: The Story of How Many
  Thousands of Men and Women Have Recovered
  from Alcoholism,* 3rd ed. New York: Alcoholics
  Anonymous World Services, Inc., 1976.

*As Bill Sees It: The A.A. Way of Life; Selected Writings
  of A.A.'s Co-founder.* New York: Alcoholics
  Anonymous World Services, Inc., 1999.

*Can A.A. Help Me Too? Black/African Americans Share
  Their Stories.* New York: Alcoholics Anonymous
  World Services, Inc., 2001.

*Daily Reflections: A Book of Reflections by A.A.
  Members for A.A. Members.* New York: Alcoholics
  Anonymous World Services, Inc., 1999.

If You Are a Professional. New York: Alcoholics
  Anonymous World Services, Inc., 1986.

Is There an Alcoholic in Your Life? New York: Alcoholics Anonymous World Services, Inc., 1976.

It Sure Beats Sitting in a Cell. New York: Alcoholics Anonymous World Services, Inc., 1979, 2000.

A Member's-Eye View of Alcoholics Anonymous. New York: Alcoholics Anonymous World Services, Inc., 1970.

Twelve Steps and Twelve Traditions: An Interpretive Commentary on the A.A. Program. New York: Alcoholics Anonymous World Services, Inc., 1999.

Twerski, Abraham J. *Waking Up Just in Time.* New York: Topper Books, 1990.

SPIRITUALITY

Fischer, Louis. *Gandhi: His Life and Message for the World.* New York: Penguin Books, 1954, 1982.

His Holiness the Dalai Lama. *How to Practice: The Way to a Meaningful Life.* Edited and translated by Jeffrey Hopkins. New York: Atria Books, 2002.

His Holiness the Dalai Lama, and Howard C. Cutler. *The Art of Happiness: A Handbook for Living.* New York: Penguin Putnam, Inc., 1998.

Kinsman Fisher, Anne. *The Legend of Tommy Morris: A Mystical Tale of True Love; Based on the True Story*

of Golf's Greatest Champion. San Rafael: Amber-
Allen Publishing, 1996.

Kinsman Fisher, Anne. *The Masters of the Spirit: A
Golf Fable*. San Francisco: Harper Collins, 1997.

Tolle, Eckhart. *The Power of Now*. Novato: New
World Library, 1999.

ABOUT THE AUTHOR

ANDREW L. DIEDEN is a recovering alcoholic and board vice president of the National Council on Alcoholism and other Drug Addictions–Bay Area (NCADA-BA). Andrew is also a UC Berkeley graduate, attorney, competitive mountain biker, and golf enthusiast. Andrew has found addiction and recovery far easier to understand and execute by relating his recovery program to the familiar language and lessons of sports. He wrote this book to help addicts and those who love them find happiness through recovery and sports. Living in northern California, Andrew has been sober eight years.

Hazelden, a national nonprofit organization founded in 1949, helps people reclaim their lives from the disease of addiction. Built on decades of knowledge and experience, Hazelden offers a comprehensive approach to addiction that addresses the full range of patient, family, and professional needs, including treatment and continuing care for youth and adults, research, higher learning, public education and advocacy, and publishing.

A life of recovery is lived "one day at a time." Hazelden publications, both educational and inspirational, support and strengthen lifelong recovery. In 1954, Hazelden published *Twenty-Four Hours a Day*, the first daily meditation book for recovering alcoholics, and Hazelden continues to publish works to inspire and guide individuals in treatment and recovery, and their loved ones. Professionals who work to prevent and treat addiction also turn to Hazelden for evidence-based curricula, informational materials, and videos for use in schools, treatment programs, and correctional programs.

Through published works, Hazelden extends the reach of hope, encouragement, help, and support to individuals, families, and communities affected by addiction and related issues.

For questions about Hazelden publications, please call **800-328-9000** or visit us online at **hazelden.org/bookstore.**

Other titles that may interest you:

My Name Is Funky . . . and I'm an Alcoholic
A Story about Alcoholism and Recovery
Tom Batiuk

My Name Is Funky follows comic strip character Funky Winkerbean's tumultuous journey and tentative recovery aided by family and friends, his AA group, and a most perceptive sponsor.

Softcover, 152 pp.   Order No. 2399

Spilled Gravy
Advice on Love, Life, and Acceptance
from a Man Uniquely Unqualified to Give It
Ed Driscoll

You will laugh out loud, wince in discomfort, and ultimately celebrate the triumph of recovery in this uproarious memoir by comedian Ed Driscoll.

Softcover, 208 pp.   Order No. 2610

When one door closes, another door opens—but it's Hell in the Hallway
Sandi Bachom

Sandi Bachom shares hundreds of witty insights she gathered in the midst of trying times in her life. The result: perspective for your journey.

Softcover, 136 pp.   Order No. 2364

Hazelden books are available at fine bookstores everywhere. To order directly from Hazelden, call 1-800-328-9000 or visit hazelden.org/bookstore.